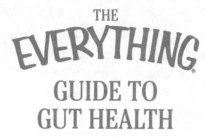

THE
EVERYTHING®
GUIDE TO
GUT HEALTH

Dear Reader,

Whether you've picked up this book to help yourself, help a family member or friend, or just to learn something new, I commend you. You have just taken one of the most important steps to improving your quality of life.

I speak to you as someone who knows the importance of having a healthy gut firsthand. I've dealt with chronic issues in my own life. It took me a long time—and many visits to the doctor—to realize that what I was dealing with all started in my gut, but as soon as I did, I took action and started making the necessary changes to fix my health.

While reading this book, you should realize that your health is in your own hands. Whether you jump right in and take every bit of advice in the book or you decide to incorporate a little bit at a time, you're moving in the right direction.

I wish you all the best in gut health and in life.

Lindsay Boyers, CHNC

Welcome to the EVERYTHING® Series!

These handy, accessible books give you all you need to tackle a difficult project, gain a new hobby, comprehend a fascinating topic, prepare for an exam, or even brush up on something you learned back in school but have since forgotten.

You can choose to read an Everything® book from cover to cover or just pick out the information you want from our four useful boxes: e-questions, e-facts, e-alerts, and e-ssentials.

We give you everything you need to know on the subject, but throw in a lot of fun stuff along the way, too.

We now have more than 400 Everything® books in print, spanning such wide-ranging categories as weddings, pregnancy, cooking, music instruction, foreign language, crafts, pets, New Age, and so much more. When you're done reading them all, you can finally say you know Everything®!

QUESTION

Answers to
common questions

FACT

Important snippets
of information

ALERT

Urgent
warnings

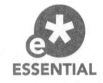

ESSENTIAL

Quick
handy tips

PUBLISHER Karen Cooper

MANAGING EDITOR, EVERYTHING® SERIES Lisa Laing

COPY CHIEF Casey Ebert

ASSISTANT PRODUCTION EDITOR Alex Guarco

ACQUISITIONS EDITOR Hillary Thompson

DEVELOPMENT EDITOR Jennifer Lawler

EVERYTHING® SERIES COVER DESIGNER Erin Alexander

Visit the entire Everything® series at www.everything.com

THE
EVERYTHING®
GUIDE TO
GUT HEALTH

- Boost Your Immune System
- Eliminate Disease
- Restore Digestive Health

Lindsay Boyers, CHNC

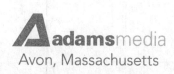

Avon, Massachusetts

To my mom, Aurora (Lola).
Thank you for always being there for me, for keeping me motivated, and for
believing in me even when I didn't believe in myself. I love you.

An Everything® Series Book.
Everything® and everything.com® are registered trademarks of F+W Media, Inc.

Published by
Adams Media, a division of F+W Media, Inc.
57 Littlefield Street, Avon, MA 02322. U.S.A.
www.adamsmedia.com

Contains material adapted and abridged from *The Everything® Mediterranean Cookbook* by Dawn Altomari-Rathjen and Jennifer Bendelius, copyright © 2003 by F+W Media, Inc., ISBN 10: 1-58062-869-9, ISBN 13: 978-1-58062-869-3; *The Everything® Food Allergy Cookbook* by Linda Larsen, copyright © 2008 by F+W Media, Inc., ISBN 10: 1-59869-560-6, ISBN 13: 978-1-59869-560-1; *The Everything® Digestive Health Book* by Angie Best-Boss with David Edelberg, copyright © 2009 by F+W Media, Inc., ISBN 10: 1-59869-959-8, ISBN 13: 978-1-59869-959-3; *The Everything® Mediterranean Diet Book* by Connie Diekman and Sam Sotiropoulos, copyright © 2010 by F+W Media, Inc., ISBN 10: 1-4405-0674-4, ISBN 13: 978-1-4405-0674-1; *The Everything® Raw Food Recipe Book* by Mike Snyder with Nancy Faass and Lorena Novak Bull, copyright © 2010 by F+W Media, Inc., ISBN 10: 1-4405-0011-8, ISBN 13: 978-1-4405-0011-4; *The Everything® Green Smoothies Book* by Britt Brandon with Lorena Novak Bull, copyright © 2011 by F+W Media, Inc., ISBN 10: 1-4405-2564-1, ISBN 13: 978-1-4405-2564-3; *The Everything® Paleolithic Diet Book* by Jodie Cohen and Gilaad Cohen, copyright © 2011 by F+W Media, Inc., ISBN 10: 1-4405-1206-X, ISBN 13: 978-1-4405-1206-3; *The Everything® Thyroid Diet Book* by Clara Schneider, copyright © 2011 by F+W Media, Inc., ISBN 10: 1-4405-1097-0, ISBN 13: 978-1-4405-1097-7; *The Everything® Coconut Diet Cookbook* by Anji Sandage with Lorena Novak Bull, copyright © 2012 by F+W Media, Inc., ISBN 10: 1-4405-2902-7, ISBN 13: 978-1-4405-2902-3; *The Everything® Eating Clean Cookbook* by Britt Brandon, copyright © 2012 by F+W Media, Inc., ISBN 10: 1-4405-2999-X, ISBN 13: 978-1-4405-2999-3; *The Everything® Giant Book of Juicing* by Teresa Kennedy, copyright © 2013 by F+W Media, Inc., ISBN 10: 1-4405-5785-3, ISBN 13: 978-1-4405-5785-9.

ISBN 10: 1-4405-8526-1
ISBN 13: 978-1-4405-8526-5
eISBN 10: 1-4405-8527-X
eISBN 13: 978-1-4405-8527-2

Printed in the United States of America.

10 9 8 7 6 5 4 3 2 1

Library of Congress Cataloging-in-Publication Data

Boyers, Lindsay.
  The everything guide to gut health / Lindsay Boyers, CHNC.
    pages cm
  Includes index.
  ISBN 978-1-4405-8526-5 (pb) -- ISBN 1-4405-8526-1 (pb) -- ISBN 978-1-4405-8527-2 (ebook) -- ISBN 1-4405-8527-X (ebook)
  1. Gastrointestinal system--Diseases--Diet therapy. 2. Cooking for the sick. I. Title.
  RC806.B69 2014
  641.5'631--dc23

                    2014033044

Many of the designations used by manufacturers and sellers to distinguish their products are claimed as trademarks. Where those designations appear in this book and F+W Media, Inc. was aware of a trademark claim, the designations have been printed with initial capital letters.

This book is intended as general information only, and should not be used to diagnose or treat any health condition. In light of the complex, individual, and specific nature of health problems, this book is not intended to replace professional medical advice. The ideas, procedures, and suggestions in this book are intended to supplement, not replace, the advice of a trained medical professional. Consult your physician before adopting any of the suggestions in this book, as well as about any condition that may require diagnosis or medical attention. The author and publisher disclaim any liability arising directly or indirectly from the use of this book.

Always follow safety and commonsense cooking protocol while using kitchen utensils, operating ovens and stoves, and handling uncooked food. If children are assisting in the preparation of any recipe, they should always be supervised by an adult.

Cover images © StockFood/Richardson, Alan; StockFood/Eising Studio-Food Photo & Video.

This book is available at quantity discounts for bulk purchases.
For information, please call 1-800-289-0963.

Contents

Acknowledgments

Thank you to my dad, Scott, who always encourages me to do better; to my sister, Tiffany, who always has my back; and to my brother, Sean, who always provides comic relief. Thank you to the rest of my family, especially my Titia Fatima, who excitedly cheers me on no matter what I'm doing. Thank you, Paul, for always making sure I'm well nourished and for keeping me on track. I love you all.

Thank you to Hillary Thompson for working alongside me from start to finish and to Jennifer Lawler for her editing expertise.

Introduction

YOUR GUT IS ITS own complex ecosystem. It's home to 100 trillion—yes, trillion—microorganisms, including about 400 different species of bacteria. The bacterial cells in your body actually outnumber the human cells. It may be unsettling to know that you're carrying around so many bugs, but they are absolutely essential to your health and your life.

Researchers have discovered that the microorganisms in the gut play crucial roles in digestion, metabolism, and immunity. Without microbes in your gut, your body couldn't break down the food you eat or use the energy it creates for body processes. Your gut is responsible for more than 75 percent of your immune system. The intestinal flora in your gut communicate with the rest of your immune system to alert your body to the presence of a potentially harmful invader.

The gut has also been nicknamed "the second brain" because it controls—at least in part—your mental state. Your gut contains 100 million neurons that respond to environmental threats, potential danger, and excitement. That's why you feel butterflies in your stomach when you're nervous or your stomach drops when you're scared. This intricate set of nerves is responsible for your "gut instincts" and subconsciously tells you how to react to environmental stimuli. Because it plays a role in so many areas of your body, a healthy gut is absolutely critical to your well-being.

If your gut is in disarray and the bacterial environment is out of balance, you're going to feel it. If you're not eliminating properly, you're going to feel it. Although digestive symptoms like bloating, gas, constipation, heartburn, diarrhea, and irritable bowel syndrome are common indicators of a damaged gut, they are only the beginning. A damaged gut is also connected to autoimmune diseases like thyroid disease, diabetes, multiple sclerosis, and lupus. Damage in your gut may be responsible for hives, skin rashes, eczema, acne, bad breath, joint pain, and muscle pain. An imbalanced gut leads to chronic fatigue and low energy levels. The list really goes on and on and on.

Unfortunately, today's modern lifestyle is toxic to your gut health. Processed foods, refined sugar, chronic stress, use of medications, and a fast-paced lifestyle have become the norm, and these are all things that can destroy your gut. Regular exposure to chemicals and toxins kills off the good bacteria in your gut and gives the bad bacteria a chance to thrive. When bad bacteria take over, your gut goes into a state of dysbiosis—or bacterial imbalance. Although you may not feel anything at first, eventually this dysbiosis can lead to uncomfortable symptoms and chronic health problems.

Fortunately, changing the way you eat and the way you live can help restore gut health and put you on the path to being the best you that you can be. If you're experiencing any chronic symptoms or health problems or you just don't feel right, then it's time to take a look at the health of your gut. It's never too late to change your life and start on the path to restoring your gut health.

CHAPTER 1

Assessing Your Gut Health

When it comes to overall wellness, maintaining your gut health is just as important as maintaining your heart health, bone health, and the health of the rest of your body. Although digestive symptoms like heartburn, gas, constipation, diarrhea, nausea, and abdominal pain are common with an unbalanced gut, they are not the only warning signs. An unhealthy gut can also present as food intolerances, skin rashes, arthritis, headaches, and chronic fatigue. Learn what normal digestive health looks like and why you shouldn't ignore those "gut feelings."

How the Digestive System Works

The food you eat is not in a form that your body can use as nourishment. It must be broken down into smaller molecules before it can be absorbed into your blood and carried to cells throughout your body. Digestion allows your body to get the nutrients and energy it needs from the food you eat. The process of digestion begins the moment you even start thinking about food.

FACT

When you see, smell, taste, or think about food, your brain sends impulses through the nerves to the salivary glands, signaling them to prepare for a meal. Your salivary glands, which are located under your lower jaw and tongue, respond by producing saliva, which helps break down food.

Parts of the Digestive System

The digestive system consists of the gastrointestinal (digestive) tract and other organs, called accessory organs, which assist in the digestion process. The digestive tract, which runs from your mouth to your anus, consists of all of the hollow organs through which food enters and then leaves your body. As food moves through the digestive tract, nutrients are extracted along the way.

Your nervous system also plays a big role in processing the food you eat. Two types of nerves, called extrinsic and intrinsic nerves, control the digestive system. Extrinsic, or outside, nerves connect to the central nervous system, which consists of the brain and spinal cord. These nerves release chemicals that tell the muscles of the digestive system to either contract or relax, depending on whether or not there is food that needs to be digested.

The intrinsic nerves are those that are inside the gastrointestinal tract. These nerves release substances that control the movement of food through the digestive tract and the production of digestive juices. The intrinsic nerves jump into action when the presence of food literally stretches the walls of the hollow organs like the stomach.

Munching Away

When you see or smell your favorite meal, your salivary glands begin to produce saliva, which contains enzymes that start to break the food into smaller components, and mucus and water, which help soften the food so that you can swallow it. When the food, now referred to as a bolus, is adequately broken down, your tongue helps move it to the back of your throat. At first, swallowing is a conscious decision, but once the swallow begins, the digestion process becomes involuntary and moves along under the control of your nerves. The esophagus, which is about 10" long, moves food from the back of your throat to your stomach.

FACT

You have a total of six salivary glands in your mouth. Approximately 99 percent of saliva is water. The rest is a mixture of enzymes and buffers that help break down your food and keep the pH in your mouth neutralized.

Muscles in the walls of the esophagus move in a wavelike motion, called peristalsis, to slowly squeeze the food along its length and down into the stomach. A muscular ring called the lower esophageal sphincter, or LES, allows food to enter the stomach and then squeezes shut to keep food or fluid from flowing back up into the esophagus. If the LES isn't working properly, stomach contents like partially digested food and stomach acid can flow backward—or reflux—into the esophagus. This is what causes acid reflux and the uncomfortable symptoms that go with it.

The Stomach's Job

The bolus travels down your esophagus until it reaches your stomach. In the stomach, the bolus comes into contact with various digestive enzymes and hydrochloric acid. The stomach muscles begin to contract and relax to mix the digestive juices with the partially digested food until it's broken down into a semi-liquid state, now referred to as chyme. The chyme makes its way through your stomach and into your small intestine, approximately 1 teaspoon at a time. An adult's stomach has a volume of just 2.5 fluid ounces when it is empty, but it can expand to hold 50 times that, or more than 100 fluid ounces, after a large meal. In someone with a healthy gut and digestive system, the total emptying of the stomach takes about 4–5 hours; however, the exact time it takes for the stomach to empty depends on the type of food being digested, the amount of fluid in it, and the health state of the gut. The more fluid present, the faster the stomach empties.

The Small Intestine

The small intestine, which is the longest part of your digestive system, does the bulk of the digestive work. Here, digestive juices from accessory organs like the liver, pancreas, and gallbladder help break down the chyme into absorbable nutrients.

The nutrients your body needs pass through the walls of your small intestine, eventually reaching the bloodstream and traveling to various cells in your body. Food matter that your body doesn't need or can't use stays inside the small intestine, where it will travel to the large intestine and eventually leave your body as waste.

Getting Rid of Waste

The undigested material from the small intestine travels to the large intestine, the body's waste-processing plant. The walls of the large intestine are smooth on the inside and house large colonies of bacteria. The bacteria act on the undigested waste and convert it into gases, acids, and vitamins. The large intestine is also responsible for absorbing excess water. The three parts of the large intestine are the cecum, the colon, and the rectum, each of which plays different roles.

FACT

The large intestine is home to the appendix, a small fingerlike pouch located near where the large and small intestine meet. It can become inflamed and extremely painful. Some scientists suggest that the appendix, once thought to be worthless, may actually produce and protect good germs in your body.

The cecum is a pouch at the beginning of the large intestine that joins the small intestine to the large intestine. This transition area expands in diameter, allowing food to travel from the small intestine to the large.

The colon connects to the rectum. It absorbs fluids and salts, and holds the resulting waste. Billions of bacteria live in the colon and help to ferment and absorb substances like fiber. If there is an imbalance in these microorganisms, it can lead to uncomfortable digestive symptoms, like gas and bloating.

The rectum is the last 12" of bowel above the anus. The rectum acts as a storage area for your feces until your next bowel movement. The anus is held closed by a ring of muscles. When you have to go to the bathroom, you relax those muscles to expel feces.

Your small intestine, which is made up of three parts, is about 20' long. Your large intestine is approximately 5' long. Although transit time varies depending on the status of your gut health and the type of food you ate, it generally takes 40–50 hours for food to travel through the entire digestive system.

The Importance of Healthy Digestion and Good Gut Health

Your body uses nutrients like vitamins, minerals, carbohydrates, protein, and fatty acids to carry out every single one of its physiological processes, such as fixing damaged cells and making new ones. Nutrients give cells what they need to work, grow, and divide. The only way to get most of the nutrients your body needs is through the foods you eat.

When your gut is healthy and your digestion is working properly, your body has access to everything it needs to keep itself healthy. When your gut is imbalanced and your digestion is out of whack, your body cannot absorb nutrients no matter how clean your diet is. Adopting a clean diet is only one aspect of gut health. You must also work to fix your damaged gut so you can absorb nutrients by taking the proper supplements, engaging in stress-reduction techniques, and staying properly hydrated.

QUESTION

What is the difference between essential and nonessential nutrients?
Essential nutrients are those that your body cannot make; therefore, you must obtain them through your diet. Nonessential nutrients are those that your body can manufacture from other chemicals and substances in your body, so it's not as vital to consume them every day, although they are just as important. Examples of nonessential nutrients include the amino acids alanine, glutamine, and arginine.

Identifying Digestive Problems

When your digestive system is working properly, you shouldn't feel any uncomfortable symptoms like bloating or belching. When the digestive system is out of balance, you may feel severe and persistent symptoms. Signs of digestive distress may include:

- Bloating, belching, burning, and flatulence after meals
- A sense of extreme fullness after eating
- Indigestion, diarrhea, or constipation
- Rectal itching
- Weak or cracked fingernails
- Dilated capillaries in the cheeks and nose
- Postadolescent acne or other skin irritations, such as rosacea, eczema, and chronic urticaria (hives)
- Iron deficiency
- Chronic intestinal infections, parasites, yeast, and unfriendly bacteria
- Greasy stools
- Easily bruised skin
- Fatigue

Figure Out Your Normal

Constipation is clinically defined as having fewer than three bowel movements per week or passing stools that are hard, dry, small, and difficult to pass; but when it comes to regularity, everyone's different. Some people have several bowel movements daily, often after each meal; others move their bowels only once per day. Your definition of constipation really depends on you and how you feel. The goal is to move your bowels at least once per day and be symptom-free—meaning no pain, abdominal discomfort, bloating, constipation sensation, or heartburn following or between meals.

FACT

Constipation affects approximately 42 million people in the United States, making it one of the most common gastrointestinal problems, according to the National Digestive Diseases Information Clearinghouse. People of any race, age, or gender can become constipated, but the condition is most common in women and adults ages 65 and older.

Signs of a poorly functioning colon include:

- Straining to pass your bowel contents
- Having a hard stool that quickly sinks to the bottom of the toilet
- Chronic diarrhea, loose stool, or constipation
- Excess gas, bloating, and abdominal cramping

Look Before You Flush

Your stool can give you clues about your overall digestive health, so peek into the toilet bowl before you flush. Healthy stool is smooth, soft, and medium to light brown in color. Your stool should come out in one piece with an ideal diameter of 1–2". Healthy stool also sinks slowly into the toilet bowl, instead of splashing noisily into the water, and doesn't have a foul odor. If your stools are hard, difficult to pass, and come out in pieces, it may be a sign of digestive trouble. Loose stools are also indicative that there's a problem with your digestion. Your stool should not float, have a repulsive odor, or contain bits of undigested food. Yellow stool may indicate a gall-bladder problem, while white or pale gray stools suggest a lack of bile. Black or bright red stools indicate bleeding in the gastrointestinal tract.

ALERT

Unless you have been chowing down on beets, the proper response to any deep red or black stools is an immediate check-in with your healthcare provider. If you have regular yellow, white, or pale gray stools, you should also make a trip to your doctor. Red or black stools can signal internal bleeding, while unusual-colored stool can indicate a serious problem with the liver or gallbladder.

Risk Factors for Digestive Problems

A number of factors affect how well your digestive system functions. Your lifestyle, including diet, exercise, smoking, and alcohol consumption, is one of the key indicators. Chronic stress also takes a toll on your digestion. For some people, chronic stress slows things down significantly. Others can't leave the bathroom during particularly stressful times. Medical history, family history, and genetics also play a role.

Just because you have one or more risk factors for digestive problems doesn't mean you will definitely develop poor digestive health. Knowing your risk factors can guide you into making the best choices for yourself, whether that means making lifestyle changes or simply being alert for any symptoms that may indicate trouble.

Journaling Foods and Symptoms

If you have digestive troubles or any symptoms that might be related to gut health, a food journal can be your best friend. Keeping track of what you eat and how your body reacts can help you identify troublesome foods or situations and allow you to take control of your digestive health.

Even people with no digestive problems can benefit from keeping a food diary for 2–3 weeks. You may be able to identify unhealthy eating patterns, such as taking in too much sugar, frequently skipping meals, or not eating enough vegetables.

ESSENTIAL

You can track your food intake the old-fashioned way—with a pen and a notebook—or you can turn to technology for an easier way to do the tracking. Many online resources offer food tracking as well as free, downloadable apps that you can carry around with you right on your cell phone.

An honest look at what you eat—and how often you eat—can be a helpful resource in choosing how to improve your diet and, as a result, your health. You may not realize that some of the foods you're eating are having a negative effect on your body until you see it on paper. Some of the foods that bother you may not bother another. For example, you may find that gluten triggers uncomfortable symptoms, while your brother, mother, or friend may have issues with dairy.

Track Food/Beverage Intake

Here are some key things to look at when tracking your intake:

- **What kind:** Track what you eat and be as specific as you can. Include the main foods from your meals as well as any beverages and condiments, like salad dressings, sour cream, and ketchup. Make a note of how the food was prepared. Did you bake your chicken or fry it? You may find that you can tolerate certain foods better when they are prepared a certain way.
- **How much:** Record the amount of food you eat. For example, list the number of items of food—say 12 pretzels—or the volume of a particular food—say ¾ cup of bran cereal. You may notice that you feel okay with a small amount of a particular food item, but larger amounts cause digestive distress.
- **Time:** Note the time of day you eat or drink. Also record what time you woke up and what time you went to bed that day so you can keep track

of how many hours pass between meals. You may notice that you have more energy if you eat breakfast within an hour of waking up or that waiting too long between meals leads to energy crashes.

Track Feelings/Activities/Company

Another important aspect of food journaling is keeping track of where you ate, your dining partners, and the mood you were in at the time.

- **Where:** It is important to note where you ate. Was it on the couch in the living room in front of the television or at the kitchen table? Did you get your meal in while you were driving in the car or at your work desk between phone calls? Tracking where you eat will help you spot unhealthy patterns that may need some adjusting.
- **The company you keep:** You may eat differently when you are with friends or family than when you are alone. Certain friends may bring out bad eating habits in you, while others help keep you on track and encourage healthy eating habits. Jot down whether you were alone or with family members or friends. List each person individually.
- **Activity:** List any activities you were doing while you were eating. Were you working, watching TV, talking on the phone, or sitting quietly? Did you take small bites and chew each one thoroughly or did you rush through your meal without thinking about it?
- **Mood:** Our moods can impact what we eat and how much. Describe how you were feeling, such as stressed, angry, worried, or excited, while you were eating. This is also a good place to note how you felt after you ate. Did you feel satisfied or overly full? Were you still hungry?

Describe and Rate Your Symptoms

List any physical symptoms you may have before, during, or after eating and then use the following scale to rate the intensity of your symptoms:

- 0 = no symptoms/not severe
- 1 = mildly severe

- 2 = moderately severe
- 3 = severe

Don't just look for immediate symptoms, like bloating or gas. Sometimes, symptoms of a food intolerance or sensitivity take hours or even days to develop. Write down any symptom that you have at any time, whether or not you think it's related to the food you're eating. This can make it easier to identify patterns and determine which foods, if any, may be causing you a problem. Pay attention to any mood changes or changes in energy levels as well. Sometimes a food sensitivity presents itself as irrational anger or extreme fatigue.

Tracking your food intake will give you insight into several aspects of your eating habits, like when you tend to crave sugar or that you're not eating close to enough vegetables. The more specific you are with tracking your intake, the more accurate your insights will be. Don't sell yourself short by neglecting to record "just a bite" here or a little sip there. In the end, you're the one who benefits from a properly tracked diet.

CHAPTER 2

Stomach Acid

You may not think about your stomach acid very often, but it's one of the most critical components of your digestive system. If you have too much or not enough stomach acid, proper digestion is nearly impossible.

The Role of Stomach Acid

Stomach acid, also called hydrochloric acid or HCl, plays a variety of roles in your body, from helping break down protein to digesting vitamins and minerals. Stomach acid activates the enzyme pepsin. Without it, your body wouldn't be able to break down proteins into their smaller components, called amino acids, which are used to build new proteins. Your body needs these proteins for practically everything it does—from hormonal signaling to immune function to nutrient transport.

Stomach acid also plays a crucial role in your immune system. Because it's so acidic, stomach acid kills any harmful bacteria, parasites, or fungi that you may ingest with contaminated food. Without adequate amounts of stomach acid, you wouldn't be able to absorb vitamin B_{12}, which is essential in proper functioning of the brain and nervous system.

FACT

Inadequate stomach acid is a common cause of vitamin B_{12} deficiency, especially in older adults. The Institute of Medicine estimates that 10–30 percent of adults over the age of fifty have difficulty absorbing the vitamin B_{12} in food due to decreased production of stomach acid. Signs of vitamin B_{12} deficiency include weakness, fatigue, lightheadedness, rapid heartbeat, pale skin, sore tongue, stomach upset, weight loss, diarrhea, constipation, and easy bruising and bleeding.

Stomach acid also plays other critical roles in the digestive process. It initiates peristalsis—the rhythmic contractions that move partially digested food from the stomach to the small intestine—and signals the pancreas to produce and release the digestive enzymes needed to finish breaking down food.

The pH of your stomach falls around 2, or very acidic, on the pH scale. The stomach protects itself from the low pH of stomach acid by secreting an alkaline, bicarbonate-based solution. The bicarbonate neutralizes the stomach acid so that it doesn't eat away its own lining.

Stomach Acid Imbalance

In a perfectly healthy gut, the stomach would produce just enough stomach acid to properly digest foods without causing any ill effects. Unfortunately, today's fast-paced lifestyle and modern diet wreak havoc on the stomach and the production of stomach acid. Some people produce too much stomach acid, while many more don't produce enough.

Overproduction of Stomach Acid

Your digestive system gets some help in breaking down food from the food itself. Most foods contain enzymes that start to digest the food before your own digestive enzymes and stomach acid take over. In a perfect world, everyone would eat whole, enzyme-rich foods and chew each bite adequately before swallowing. Doing so ensures that the food entering your stomach contains all the enzymes necessary to help predigest your food, breaking down a large portion of your food before your stomach acid even gets involved. Unfortunately, the opposite usually happens.

FACT

The International Foundation for Functional Gastrointestinal Disorders reports that 44 percent of Americans have heartburn at least once a month, while 7 percent experience it daily. Heartburn is the most common symptom of gastroesophageal reflux disease, a condition whose prevalence is rapidly increasing worldwide.

Most food is cooked before eating. The cooking process destroys nearly all of the enzymes in the food before it even enters your mouth. If you're cooking processed food, the news is even worse. Like cooking, processing destroys the live enzymes in the food. When you eat enzyme-deficient food, the food just sits in your stomach without any predigestion taking place. If you've ever felt like there was a lump or brick in your stomach after eating, this is why.

In an attempt to compensate for the lack of enzymes present, your stomach produces an excess amount of stomach acid. Your pancreas also responds by dumping increasing amounts of enzymes into your small intestine. Instead of solving the problem, however, this leads to other problems, like gas, bloating, heartburn, indigestion, and chronic digestive disorders.

Over time, the overstimulation of the pancreas can actually lead to decreased function. The pancreas becomes overtaxed and stops producing enough digestive enzymes to make proper digestion possible. When symptoms develop, your first instinct may be to reach for an antacid pill or ask your doctor for a prescription to decrease stomach acid, but again, this only exacerbates the problem. While an antacid may diminish symptoms in the short-term, it does nothing to fix the underlying digestive issue causing the symptoms in the first place and may actually lead to low stomach acid, a much more common issue.

ALERT

Acid-neutralizing medications work in a variety of ways, but they all share one main goal: to reduce or eliminate stomach acid. This seems like a good thing, especially when you're in the throes of heartburn, but these medications do nothing to treat the underlying cause of your digestive issues and can eventually cause your stomach to stop producing enough hydrochloric acid.

Not Enough Stomach Acid

Although many physicians are quick to point the finger at excess stomach acid as the cause of many digestive issues, it's low stomach acid, or hypochlorhydria, that's the bigger issue.

Several problems can cause your body to stop producing adequate amounts of stomach acid.

- Vitamin and mineral deficiencies
- Chronic stress
- Overgrowth of bacteria, especially *Helicobacter pylori* (*H. pylori*) in the stomach

- Overgrowth of yeast like *Candida albicans*
- Chronic use of antacids, proton pump inhibitors, or H2 receptor antagonists
- Advancing age (a 60-year-old generally produces 75 percent less hydrochloric acid than a 20-year-old)

Effects of Low Stomach Acid

An inability to produce adequate amounts of stomach acid is not just uncomfortable, it can also lead to serious health consequences. Stomach acid must be present in order for your body to absorb many nutrients, including vitamin B_{12}, folic acid, copper, zinc, calcium, iron, and protein.

Stomach acid is also a vital component of your immune system. Stomach acid acts as a harsh barrier that kills any potentially harmful bacteria or parasites that enter the stomach. Without adequate amounts of stomach acid, you become susceptible to bacterial imbalances. The longer you go without producing adequate amounts of stomach acid, the greater your risk of nutritional deficiencies and bacterial imbalance becomes.

FACT

Stomach acid has a pH of around 2. When stomach acid is diminished, the pH of your stomach can increase to 4–5. It is at this pH level that bacterial overgrowth typically occurs.

Without adequate amounts of stomach acid, it's also nearly impossible to properly digest your food. Stomach acid directly breaks down food and the low pH of stomach acid activates pepsin, the enzyme needed to break down proteins. A lack of stomach acid results in partially digested food, which causes a host of issues like gas, bloating, heartburn, chronic belching, diarrhea, constipation, skin diseases, and autoimmune disorders. Low stomach acid is also associated with chronic intestinal disorders like Crohn's disease and irritable bowel syndrome and the development of food intolerances.

Signs of Low Stomach Acid

Low stomach acid can cause a wide range of symptoms and issues that can vary significantly from person to person; however, there are a few signs that seem to be the most common in people who are experiencing an underproduction of stomach acid. It may seem counterintuitive, but a large indicator of low stomach acid is frequently experiencing acid reflux after eating a meal. The problems associated with low stomach acid can lead to an increase in pressure in your abdomen. If the pressure becomes too great, the lower esophageal sphincter opens when it's not supposed to, allowing stomach acid to flow backward into your esophagus. When the stomach acid comes into contact with the inner surface of your esophagus, which doesn't have a protective lining like your stomach, it results in the characteristic pain and burning associated with heartburn.

ALERT

If heartburn seems worse than usual or is accompanied by shortness of breath, dizziness, nausea, sweating, or pain that travels into your shoulder or arm, seek emergency medical help. These symptoms may indicate a heart attack.

Many people belch or pass gas after eating a meal, but these digestive symptoms aren't normal; in fact, they're usually a sign of low stomach acid production. If you experience bloating or gas within a couple hours after eating, or you have a heavy feeling in your stomach like your food is sitting there stagnant, you may have low stomach acid. Another indicator is feeling bad or "heavy" after eating a protein-rich meal. If you don't have enough stomach acid, your body can't use pepsin properly and, as a result, proteins remain partially undigested and sit in your stomach longer than they should.

Testing for Low Stomach Acid

If you suspect your stomach acid levels are low, there are a few at-home tests you can do to prove or disprove your theory. These tests aren't scientific, but they can give you some direction for what to do next.

The first test is the baking soda test. When you get up in the morning, before you eat or drink anything else, drink a mixture of ¼ teaspoon of baking soda and 1 cup of water. When baking soda comes into contact with stomach acid, it reacts by forming carbon dioxide gas. The result is burping. If you haven't burped within 2–3 minutes of downing the baking soda mixture, it's likely that you have low stomach acid. Repeat this test over the course of the next 2 days to be sure.

Another at-home test you can do to check for low stomach acid levels is the betaine hydrochloride test. Betaine is available in supplement form. If you have normal levels of stomach acid, you should feel a warm sensation in your stomach area after taking just one of these supplements. If you have low stomach acid, it typically takes more than one. To do the test, purchase a quality betaine HCl supplement that contains 650 mg per capsule. On day 1, take 1 supplement right before each large meal. On day 2, take 2 supplements before each meal. Increase the amount of supplements you take before each meal—up to 10 days and 10 tablets—until you feel the warmth. The more supplements you have to take until you feel that warmth, the more likely you are to have low levels of stomach acid.

If you've done the at-home tests for stomach acid and you suspect that you're dealing with an underproduction of stomach acid, you can ask your doctor for the Heidelberg stomach acid test. The test is more costly—usually ranging from $300–$350—but it will give you exact results that are scientifically proven. During the test, you swallow a small capsule that contains a pH meter and a radio transmitter, then drink a solution of sodium bicarbonate (the same ingredient in baking soda). During this time, you're hooked up to a machine that measures the pH of your stomach. Once the results are printed, your doctor can determine what kind of stomach acid problems you're dealing with.

For accurate test results, fast for 8–12 hours prior to taking the Heidelberg test. You must not take proton pump inhibitors or any over-the-counter antacids or medications for at least 5 days prior to the test. Get specific recommendations for coming off any medications from your doctor.

Correcting Stomach Acid Problems

So you've determined that you have a stomach acid imbalance: now what? The ultimate goal is to restore your health to optimal levels so that supplementation is not necessary, but this process takes time. Until then, there are a number of things you can do to help your body balance stomach acid production so that you're able to properly digest food.

Acid Supplementation

When your stomach is not producing enough stomach acid, you need to give your body the acid it needs through supplements. Taking the betaine HCl supplements that you used for the at-home stomach acid tests regularly can help boost stomach acid and get digestion working again.

Figuring Out Your Dose

If your stomach is really low in stomach acid, taking one HCl tablet here and there isn't only a waste of time, it's also a waste of money. In order for the HCl supplements to work, you have to do some trial and error to figure out your correct dosage. Take one HCl tablet (650 mg or less), then eat a protein-rich meal, one that contains around 6 ounces of meat. Once you've finished your meal, pay attention to any signs of digestive distress. If you feel warmth, burning, or a feeling of heaviness after taking just one pill, it's likely that low stomach acid is not your issue. If you don't experience any of these symptoms, you'll need to do some self-experimentation to figure out your dose.

Take 2 pills before each meal for the entire next day. After each meal, pay attention for any warmth, like the feeling you get when you drink a hot beverage. The goal is to find the number of pills that make you feel that warmth and then scale back by one, so if you experience warmth after 2 pills, you'll know that your correct dose is one pill before each meal. If you don't feel anything, continue the process, increasing your dosage by 1 pill per day, until you feel that warmth.

ALERT

You should not feel any extreme discomfort when taking hydrochloric acid supplements. If you experience intense burning, stop taking them right away. If you have peptic ulcers or a history of peptic ulcers, do not supplement with betaine HCl. Do not take hydrochloric acid supplements with nonsteroidal anti-inflammatory drugs. Doing so can damage the lining of the gastrointestinal tract and increase the risk of developing a stomach ulcer.

Don't be alarmed if you need 5 or 6 pills in the beginning. It's important to give your body the amount it needs to help restore gut function. As your stomach acid production increases, the amount of supplementation you need usually lessens. The amount of time it takes depends on your gut health, but it could be weeks, months, or years. Patience and consistency are key. If you've been taking 5 pills per meal for 6 months and then all of a sudden you start to feel increased warmth at that dose, you'll know it's time to reduce the amount of pills you take. It's extremely beneficial to work with a qualified health professional who can help you figure out your correct dosage and when to reduce intake.

Digestive Enzymes

Unless you're following a raw diet, your body may be lacking some of the enzymes needed to break down the food you're eating. Even if there are adequate amounts of enzymes present, many of them are useless unless they're activated by stomach acid. You can help digestion along by taking digestive enzymes in addition to betaine HCl supplements. Some HCl supplements even contain pepsin or a variety of digestive enzymes in one tablet to make things easier and more cost-effective. When taking digestive enzymes, follow the manufacturer's instructions on the label for the correct amount.

Raw Apple Cider Vinegar

You can use raw apple cider vinegar as a quick fix for stomach acid problems as you work to correct the condition long-term. Apple cider vinegar is acidic, so it lowers the pH in the stomach, helping you digest your food more easily. Apple cider vinegar may also help correct the overgrowth of *Candida*, which can contribute to the development of low stomach acid in the first place.

If you experience heartburn after meals, raw apple cider vinegar works as a quick solution because the low pH signals the lower esophageal sphincter to close tightly, stopping the backflow of stomach contents into the esophagus. To be effective, apple cider vinegar must be raw with the "mother" intact. The "mother" is a ball of living enzymes and nutrients that are responsible for many of the vinegar's health benefits. You can tell if the mother is intact just by looking at the bottle—it is a floating web-like structure that makes the vinegar appear murky and cloudy.

Mix 1 teaspoon of raw apple cider vinegar with 4 ounces of water and drink the mixture upon waking. Repeat this process before each meal and after a meal if you experience heartburn.

Dietary Changes

Taking supplements to help correct stomach acid production is a good start, but to maximize the effectiveness of these supplements, you need to change your diet and dietary habits, too. One of the most important things you can do is mentally prepare your body for digestion before each meal. This may seem silly, but when you're stressed, your body may produce too much or too little stomach acid. Eat meals in a relaxed state. Sit down for meals, keep away from distractions like your cell phone and television, chew slowly and carefully, and savor each bite.

When you're working to correct your stomach acid levels, avoid grain products, like cereals and bread, which contain a compound called phytic acid. Phytic acid not only inhibits the action of the enzymes that are necessary for proper digestion, but it's also quick to bind with other minerals, like calcium, magnesium, iron, and zinc, making them unavailable for absorption in your body. It's best to eliminate grains from the diet, at least until your stomach acid levels return to normal, but if you don't want to do that, soak grains in a mixture of 1 teaspoon of lemon juice or apple cider vinegar per 1 cup of warm water overnight before eating them.

FACT

It takes about 20 minutes after you start eating for the brain to register if you're full. If you're not paying attention while you eat—like when eating while watching television—you don't process that information as well and you're more likely to overeat.

You can reduce stomach acid production by removing spicy foods, salty foods, and acidic foods, like citrus fruits, from your diet. These foods contribute to excess stomach acid.

A Word on Hydration

There's no doubt about it: water is important; but it's possible to be too hydrated, especially during mealtimes. If your stomach acid production is low, the last thing you want to do is dilute the stomach acid you do have even further by drinking water with your meals. Drink water at least 30 minutes before meals or 30–60 minutes after meals. If you feel as though you must have something to quench your thirst during a meal, turn to warm homemade bone broth, which is full of gelatin and can help stimulate digestive juices. Another option is to drink a small amount of raw homemade yogurt during meals. Homemade yogurt not only contains vital enzymes, but it also provides probiotics that can help balance the bacteria in your gut.

Ditch the Meds

Nonsteroidal anti-inflammatory drugs, or NSAIDS, can stimulate the body's production of stomach acid and contribute to the development of ulcers. If you have any symptoms that indicate your body may be producing too much stomach acid, avoid taking NSAIDS.

CHAPTER 3

Food Intolerances, Sensitivities, and Allergies

Many people who have a reaction to food are quick to classify that reaction as a food allergy, but there's a big difference between an allergy, which can be life-threatening, and a sensitivity or an intolerance, which can cause similar symptoms to an allergy, but do not cause an immediate life-threatening reaction.

What's the Difference?

A true food allergy involves an immune response that affects several organs in your body. If you're allergic to a certain food—say peanuts—even a minuscule amount of that food can cause an immediate, severe reaction. When you're exposed to a food you're allergic to for the first time, your body mistakenly identifies that food as a harmful substance, triggering an immune response. The immune system attempts to attack and neutralize that substance by releasing antibodies to fight it. The next time even a tiny amount of that food enters your body, your body creates an inflammatory response. Food allergies can range from mild to severe.

The most common food allergy symptoms include:

- Tingling or itching in the mouth
- Hives
- Itchiness
- Swelling of the lips, face, tongue, or throat
- Swelling of other areas of the body
- Wheezing or trouble breathing
- Nasal congestion
- Abdominal pain or diarrhea
- Nausea or vomiting
- Dizziness, lightheadedness, or fainting

A life-threatening allergic reaction is called anaphylaxis. Symptoms of anaphylaxis can include:

- Tightening of airways
- Swollen throat
- Difficulty breathing
- Rapid pulse
- Dizziness or loss of consciousness
- Severe drop in blood pressure

Eight foods are responsible for 90 percent of all allergic reactions. These foods include peanuts, tree nuts, milk, eggs, soy, wheat, fish, and shellfish.

Even a minuscule amount of these foods can produce a reaction in someone who's allergic.

ALERT

True food allergies affect only 1–4 percent of the population, while food sensitivities are much more common—and on the rise due to the increasing number of people who experience problems with gut health.

The terms *food intolerance* and *food sensitivity* are often used interchangeably, but they're not actually the same thing. A food intolerance, such as lactose intolerance, occurs when a person lacks a specific enzyme to digest a particular food item. Without the enzyme, consuming the food will produce a gastrointestinal response, not an immune system response. Although symptoms of a food intolerance are uncomfortable, they are not immediately dangerous. If you are intolerant to a certain food, you may even be able to eat small amounts of the food without experiencing any symptoms.

QUESTION

What is one of the main differences between a food allergy and a food sensitivity or intolerance?
One of the easiest ways to tell the difference is in the amount of time it takes to display symptoms. A true allergy shows symptoms very quickly, usually within an hour, while a food sensitivity or intolerance may take a few hours to days to present. This can make it difficult to spot a food sensitivity.

Possible symptoms of a food intolerance include:

- Stomach pain
- Gas and bloating
- Nausea and vomiting
- Heartburn
- Diarrhea

- Headaches
- Irritability and anxiety

Like a food allergy, a food sensitivity involves the immune system, but it produces a milder, delayed response. Symptoms of a food sensitivity may include abdominal cramps, nausea, and acid reflux. The symptoms you experience may even be different every time you're exposed to the food.

A food sensitivity may also develop due to repeated exposure to a specific food. If you eat eggs for breakfast every single day for years, you're more likely to develop sensitivity to them than if you switched up your breakfast meal.

Common Food Offenders

Some food offenders can be tough to identify because the food may be found in various types of products. Corn, for example, can appear not only in corn flakes or canned corn, but might also sweeten packaged foods in the form of high-fructose corn syrup. You may become sensitive to preservatives and additives found in processed and packaged food. For example, inulin is an additive made of fruit residues that can be found in butter, ice cream, yogurt, cereals, and jams.

Other common food triggers include:

- Artificial additives (MSG, coloring)
- Artificial sweeteners
- Citrus
- Coffee and caffeine
- Corn and corn derivatives
- Dairy products
- Eggs
- Gluten
- Peanuts and tree nuts
- Shellfish
- Soy
- Wheat and refined flour

Food Allergy Treatments

There is no way to cure a food allergy; however, some food allergies go away with time. The only way to avoid symptoms is to remove the food to which you are allergic from your diet. If you experience symptoms of anaphylaxis (serious allergic response), such as wheezing and swelling of the lips or throat, seek emergency medical care.

ALERT

If you or someone in your family has a severe food allergy, you may want to consider purchasing Food Allergy Restaurant Cards to share at restaurants you frequent, which explain the food allergy, warn about cross-contamination, list potentially dangerous foods and ingredients, and tell when to call 911.

On the other hand, you can minimize or eliminate some food sensitivities by correcting the underlying problem causing the sensitivity. In many cases, an unhealthy gut is to blame for the development of both food intolerances and sensitivities. If your gut is unhealthy, you may even experience a sensitivity to more than one food.

Testing for Food Allergies, Intolerances, and Sensitivities

To help determine if you're dealing with a food allergy, intolerance, or sensitivity, you can take several different tests. Some take very little time (such as a blood test) while others require a bigger commitment on your part (such as an elimination diet).

Whether you opt for blood tests, skin tests, or elimination diets, you can begin to identify the culprits in your diet causing you grief. Very few skin tests work for food sensitivities, but you may find that a combination of dietary changes and diagnostic tests give you the answers you're seeking.

Blood and Skin Tests

With true food allergies, it's easier to identify the offending food because the reaction occurs so quickly. To diagnose a food allergy, your physician will ask you for a thorough medical history and then conduct a series of tests like a skin prick test, a blood test, an oral food challenge, and a trial elimination diet.

Because the symptoms of food intolerances and sensitivities may occur hours to days after eating the offending food, these are much harder to diagnose. Screening blood tests, which check for up to 100 commonly eaten foods, can be helpful, but the most valuable diagnostic tool is a food sensitivity elimination diet. Your doctor can order food sensitivity blood tests, as well as tests to check for lactose intolerance and gluten sensitivity.

Elimination Diet

Various elimination diets work differently to identify problematic foods. Regardless of what approach you try, keep an accurate food journal for the time period you are testing. Do not try to rely solely on your memory.

ESSENTIAL

If you're going to follow an elimination diet, make sure to commit to at least 21 days. This is the amount of time it takes to clear your system of any potentially bothersome food or additives. Many health experts recommend following a strict elimination diet for 30 days.

The most comprehensive elimination diet involves completely removing all foods most likely to cause a reaction for 30 days. This includes dairy, eggs, corn, grains, citrus, nuts, seeds, shellfish, and soy products. Elimination diets also require you to remove processed foods that contain chemicals and artificial ingredients. If you feel exactly the same after one month of strict elimination, with absolutely no improvement of your symptoms, then food intolerances or sensitivities may not be present. If you notice fewer symptoms or an improvement in severity of symptoms, you may be on to something. Now it's time to play detective and identify exactly which foods are causing your problems.

The day after your elimination diet is complete, pick one food group to add back into your diet. You may choose any of the food groups you wish, but it's important to include only one at a time so you can single it out if a reaction occurs. If you choose dairy, have a glass of milk in the morning, butter on your veggies at lunch, and some cottage cheese with dinner. Continue this process for the next 48 hours, with the same food group, and record any symptoms, or lack thereof, in your journal. Even if you think a symptom is unrelated to your diet, write it down. You may notice patterns that point to a possible food sensitivity. Once you've discovered how that food group affects you, go back on your elimination diet for 24 hours and then redo the process with another food group.

This is when you get to make educated decisions regarding your diet and your health. If a food group gives you any type of reaction, whether it's mild or severe, it's likely that you're sensitive to that food. At this point, the best decision would be to eliminate that food from your diet, at least until your gut is repaired. In some cases, you may be able to eliminate all or some food sensitivities once your gut is restored and go back to enjoying those foods in moderation.

Gluten Sensitivities

When it comes to food sensitivities, gluten—a protein found in wheat, barley, and rye—is a major culprit. Gluten sensitivities are broken down into two major categories, celiac disease and gluten sensitivity, depending on how the body responds to the protein. Celiac disease, which involves an immune reaction to gluten, is the more serious of the two.

Celiac Disease

The Mayo Clinic describes celiac disease, which is four times more common now than it was six decades ago, as a major public health issue. It is estimated that celiac disease affects approximately 1 in 100 people, although the Celiac Disease Foundation estimates that 2.5 million people remain undiagnosed. In those who have celiac disease, the consumption of gluten triggers an immune response. The immune system sends out antibodies that attack the small intestine. This attack damages the small fingerlike projections, called villi, that line the inner surface of the small intestine. When the villi are damaged, they cannot absorb nutrients properly. Over time, unmanaged celiac disease can lead to nutritional deficiencies and long-term health complications, such as anemia, osteoporosis, infertility, and migraines.

Symptoms of celiac disease include:

- Abdominal bloating
- Pain
- Diarrhea or constipation
- Vomiting
- Weight loss
- Foul-smelling stool
- Fatigue
- Joint pain
- Depression or anxiety
- Missed periods
- Tingling or numbness in the hands and feet
- Canker sores
- Itchy skin or rash

Gluten Sensitivity

Gluten sensitivity is a condition similar to celiac disease, although it's not as severe. Those who are sensitive to gluten experience symptoms after eating the protein, but no damage to the villi in the small intestine occurs. If you have non-celiac gluten sensitivity, you may experience depression, difficulty concentrating, abdominal pain, bloating, diarrhea, and a foggy head.

Finding Relief

Whether you have celiac disease or gluten sensitivity, the treatment is the same: avoid eating any foods that contain gluten. With the rise in gluten-sensitive individuals also came a rise in processed and packaged gluten-free foods. While these items are technically "safe" for a gluten-free diet, they are often not the best choice. Many gluten-free products contain other potentially problematic foods, like soy and milk. The best way to follow a gluten-free diet is to choose whole foods that are naturally gluten-free. Fill up your plate with a colorful array of fresh vegetables and some grilled meat, and eat plenty of healthy fats like avocado and coconut oil.

ESSENTIAL

Current research estimates that approximately 18 million Americans have gluten sensitivity. This is about 6 times the amount of people who have celiac disease. While a doctor can diagnose celiac disease with a blood test, non-celiac gluten sensitivity does not show up in the same way. The best way to figure out if you are sensitive to gluten is through a special antibody testing or an elimination diet.

If you have celiac disease, it may not be enough just to take gluten out of your diet. The protein is often found in medications, cosmetics, and household items, meaning you could inadvertently ingest a small amount, so diligently check labels before you buy. Manufacturers can change ingredients without warning, so don't assume something is gluten-free just because you've purchased it before. Check labels every time you purchase a product, even if it's a familiar one.

Other products that may contain gluten include:

- Lipstick/lip balm
- Sunscreen
- Children's stickers and price tags
- Stamps and envelopes
- Washing machine detergent
- Soaps and shampoos
- Toothpaste and mouthwash
- Cosmetics

Eating Out Gluten-Free

Many restaurants offer gluten-free menus. With the rising prevalence of celiac disease and gluten sensitivity, most restaurants are willing to accommodate a gluten-free diner even if they don't have a specified gluten-free menu. Call ahead and speak to a manager if you're not sure. Make your dieting restrictions clear and ask any questions you have. Don't assume just because a food, like meat, is naturally gluten-free that it's a safe choice. Many restaurants coat meat in flour to make it crispier or add bread crumbs to meatballs to help them stick together. They may also add flour to thicken sauces or gravies. Don't be afraid to ask questions.

Lactose Intolerance

Lactose intolerance is a condition in which your body can't properly digest the milk sugar lactose. One type of lactose intolerance occurs because of damage to the gut, and may only be temporary, reversing when the gut is fully healed.

As you age, your body's production of lactase, the enzyme needed to digest the milk sugar lactose, gradually decreases, which causes some people to develop lactose intolerance. If you're lactose intolerant, your body will let you know in the form of stomach cramps and diarrhea 30 minutes to 2 hours after your ice cream sundae.

Other symptoms of lactose intolerance include:

- Abdominal bloating
- Gas
- Stomach cramps
- Flatulence
- Diarrhea
- Bad breath (generally much worse than typical morning breath and resistant to good oral hygiene)

Lactose Intolerance Versus Dairy Allergy

Lactose intolerance differs from a dairy allergy in several ways. Adults are more likely to be lactose intolerant, while a dairy allergy often occurs in infants and is usually outgrown by the age of two or three. The most common symptoms of lactose intolerance are stomach cramps and diarrhea; a dairy allergy usually causes rashes, hives, vomiting, or diarrhea. If you're lactose intolerant, the milk sugar lactose is to blame for your symptoms; with a dairy allergy, the culprit is either casein or whey, the two proteins in milk.

Management Strategies

Lactose intolerance may be inconvenient, but it can be managed. To avoid the symptoms of lactose intolerance, remove anything that contains lactose from your diet. It sounds simple enough—get rid of milk and milk products, like ice cream, yogurt, and cheese—but it's not that easy. Many packaged foods contain lactose, and it often sneaks into a food product under a different name.

ALERT

Grocery items that may contain lactose include processed and prepared foods such as bread, baked goods, candy, cookies, breakfast drinks, chocolate drink mixes, sauces and gravies, frosting, frozen dinners, pancake and biscuit mixes, coffee creamer, and snack foods.

Some people with lactose intolerance may not be able to have any dairy at all, while others do okay with a low level of lactose. Once you have identified lactose as a problem for you, remove any lactose-containing products from your diet for several weeks. Gradually increase the amount of lactose you eat to see how much you can tolerate, if any. Start with a small amount, like a tablespoon of milk or a small chunk of cheese. Every couple of days, double the amount you take in until you reach your tolerance. Fermented milk products such as yogurt, containing *L. bulgaricus* and *S. thermophilus*, may help decrease the symptoms of lactose intolerance and seem to be tolerated fairly well by most people who are lactose intolerant.

Getting Calcium

If you need to restrict your dairy consumption, you're probably wondering how you'll meet your calcium needs. Fortunately, there are many calcium-rich choices that don't contain dairy. Sardines and canned pink salmon with the bones are two of the richest sources of nondairy calcium. Other options include collard greens, spinach, turnip greens, kale, okra, dandelion greens, blue crab, and clams.

CHAPTER 4

Recognizing Leaky Gut

Leaky gut has been getting a lot of attention in the alternative health community recently, and for good reason. Leaky gut is the name given to a condition characterized by increased intestinal permeability. In someone with leaky gut, substances that normally wouldn't be able to pass through the small intestine do. Leaky gut is associated with a wide range of health issues from food allergies and intolerance to hyperactivity to skin conditions, like psoriasis, eczema, and acne. A common misconception is that if you're not experiencing any digestive distress, your gut is in good health. This couldn't be further from the truth—especially in the case of leaky gut.

Leaky Gut Basics

Your intestinal lining is one of the first lines of defense for your immune system. Your small intestine has the tough job of deciding what's safe to enter the blood and what may be hazardous to your health and needs to be eliminated through your digestive tract. In a healthy gut, nothing can pass through the lining into the bloodstream without the "okay" that it's safe.

FACT

Because the small intestine allows some things to pass into the bloodstream, while blocking out others, it's classified as semipermeable. In someone with leaky gut, the small intestine transitions into a permeable membrane. A permeable membrane allows all substances to pass through without discrimination.

When someone has leaky gut, the previously tight junctions between cells become loose and instead of blocking toxins and undigested material from passing through the intestinal lining into the blood, the small intestine allows nearly everything to pass through. Because these large, undigested molecules and toxic materials aren't supposed to be in the blood, your body recognizes them as hazardous and sends out a red alert.

The first to respond is your liver, whose job is to filter out any potential toxins or hazardous materials that make it past your small intestine.

In someone with a healthy gut, the liver may have only a few things to filter here and there; in someone with leaky gut, there is so much waste and undigested food particles making their way into the blood that the liver is unable to keep up and calls on the immune system for backup.

FACT

Your liver is your biggest detoxification organ. The liver is responsible for processing all of the food you eat. It also removes toxins, smoke, and chemicals from the air that you breathe in. When you're exposed to too many toxins, the liver can become overloaded. When this happens, it doesn't function as well as it as should and toxins are left in the body.

The immune system goes on the attack by sending out antibodies in an attempt to neutralize the food particles. Next time these food particles enter the bloodstream, your immune system may recognize them as an allergy or sensitivity and react accordingly. The problem isn't just that having increased intestinal permeability makes you more susceptible to the development of food sensitivities, intolerances, and allergies; the antibodies also attack the healthy cells, which can lead to widespread inflammation. Inflammation causes a great deal of stress on your system and can make leaky gut even worse.

Causes of Leaky Gut

Many health experts agree that certain factors, such as the kinds of food you eat, stress, and toxins in your environment, contribute to the development of leaky gut. Each factor leads to inflammation, the underlying cause of increased intestinal permeability.

QUESTION

Is inflammation always bad?
No, inflammation is not always a bad thing. In fact, inflammation is a necessary part of the immune response. Inflammation helps protect the body from injury and infection and helps the wound-healing process. When inflammation is chronic or long-lasting, however, it can put a great deal of stress on the body and eventually lead to chronic disease.

The key to getting rid of leaky gut and restoring the integrity of your small intestine is to find out what factor or factors are contributing to chronic inflammation and remove them.

The Food You Eat

Your diet plays a large role in the development of leaky gut. When you consume a large amount of processed foods, refined grains and sugars, preservatives, and artificial flavorings and colorings, you expose your small intestine to a huge amount of chemicals that it doesn't recognize as food.

Because your small intestine doesn't really know how to process this matter, toxins accumulate. This leads to inflammation, which can destroy the lining of your gut. Unknowingly consuming foods that you are sensitive, intolerant, or allergic to, such as in the case of undiagnosed celiac disease, also plays a role in the development of leaky gut.

The Stress You're Under

Chronic stress is just as dangerous to the body as an unhealthy diet. When you're under a great deal of stress, your immune system becomes suppressed. A suppressed immune system cannot protect the body as well as a healthy immune system. The result is widespread inflammation that leads to increased gut permeability.

Infections and Toxins

Infections that can contribute to leaky gut include intestinal parasites and small intestinal bacterial overgrowth (SIBO). Yeast, which is a part of the normal flora in your gut, can get out of hand, as in the case of *Candida* overgrowth, and cause damage to the small intestine, contributing to holes in its lining.

FACT

Small intestinal bacterial overgrowth (SIBO) may be an underlying cause of irritable bowel syndrome and Crohn's disease. It's also common in many autoimmune diseases, including celiac disease, Hashimoto's disease, and scleroderma.

In someone with SIBO, large numbers of bacteria from the large intestine make their way into the small intestine. When bacterial numbers get too high, they begin to produce toxins, enzymes, and gases that disrupt normal digestion and damage the lining of the small intestine. Someone with SIBO may experience excessive gas, bloating, constipation, diarrhea, and abdominal pain in addition to related chronic health problems. Sustained exposure to toxins, like medications, mercury, pollution, and chemicals, to name a few, can also damage the intestinal lining and contribute to leaky gut.

Signs of Leaky Gut

Symptoms and signs of leaky gut vary widely from person to person. The following signs are some of the ones most commonly associated with leaky gut:

- Multiple food sensitivities
- Digestive issues like gas, bloating, constipation, or diarrhea
- Seasonal allergies or respiratory problems like asthma
- The presence of autoimmune diseases including, but not limited to, rheumatoid arthritis, Hashimoto's disease, or lupus
- Nutritional deficiencies
- Skin rashes
- Recurring sickness or infection
- Hormonal imbalances
- Diagnosis of chronic fatigue syndrome or fibromyalgia
- Mood and behavioral issues like anxiety, depression, or ADHD
- Headaches, brain fog, and memory loss

Leaky Gut and Autoimmune Diseases

According to the American Autoimmune Related Diseases Association, there are 80–100 identified autoimmune diseases and an additional 40 diseases with an autoimmune component. The prevalence of autoimmune diseases is rising rapidly and no part of your body is, well, immune. Autoimmune diseases can affect your heart, lungs, skin, nervous system, and endocrine system, which controls your hormones, to name a few. Previously, researchers were stumped as to what causes some people to develop autoimmune diseases while others don't. Current research shows that the development of autoimmune diseases may start in the gut.

If you've been diagnosed with an autoimmune disease, asking your doctor for additional laboratory testing can help determine whether or not intestinal permeability may play a role in the cause of the disease. Your doctor can test for celiac disease through blood testing and SIBO through a non-invasive breath test.

The test for SIBO is called the hydrogen breath test. At the beginning of the test, you blow a breath of air into a balloon and then consume a small amount of sugar, usually glucose or lactulose. Every 15 minutes after you ingest the test sugar, your breath will be tested for hydrogen and methane. The amount of gas in your breath can tell your doctor if there is an overgrowth of bacteria in your small intestine.

Normally, there is no gas in the breath because the sugar never reaches the gas-producing bacteria that usually live only in the colon. If there is gas in the breath, it indicates that the bacteria have made their way to the small intestine where they are exposed to the sugar, which they feed on.

Three Factors of Autoimmunity

Dr. Alessio Fasano, a pediatric gastroenterologist and research scientist, believes that all autoimmune diseases share three common characteristics: a genetic predisposition, exposure to an environmental trigger, and some degree of intestinal permeability, or leaky gut. In the February 2012 issue of *Clinical Reviews in Allergy & Immunology* Dr. Fasano reports that contrary to popular belief, the autoimmune process could be stopped, and possibly reversed, by fixing leaky gut.

Individuals who are genetically predisposed to autoimmune diseases seem to have irregularities in what is called the zonulin system. Zonulin is a substance normally present in the intestines. This substance controls which fluids, molecules, and cells pass through the intestinal barrier.

In people with autoimmune conditions, zonulin seems to be overexpressed, which means that it lets too many things pass through the small intestine and doesn't block out enough. Some studies have shown that this process may be involved in many autoimmune conditions, including type 1 diabetes, celiac disease, and multiple sclerosis.

Restoring Gut Integrity

Restoring gut integrity is a multifaceted approach that involves diet changes, lifestyle modifications, and proper supplementation. The key is to remove any toxic triggers from your body, while giving your body the nutrients it needs to restore the intestinal lining. The most common approach to correcting leaky gut in the world of functional medicine is called the Four "R" Approach. The four R's of this program are remove, replace, reinoculate, and repair.

Remove

As the name suggests, the remove portion of the program requires you to remove all of the things that cause damage to your gut. This includes toxic organisms, like bacteria, parasites, and yeast, as well as toxic molecules like hormones, antibiotics, preservatives, and chemical additives, many of which are found in your food. While you can remove toxic and inflammatory foods on your own, you may need the help of a functional medicine doctor to determine the presence of any underlying infections.

"Remove" also applies to chronic stress or stressful situations. Everyone deals with stress at some point and it's unrealistic—read: impossible—to try to remove all stress from your life, but the key is to find healthy ways to deal with it so that it doesn't become a chronic problem that taxes your system. Practice meditation or take a yoga class. Put the computer away and get lost in a book. Spend some time doing something that you really love, like drawing or writing. Just make sure to spend some time in your happy place, wherever that may be.

Changing Your Diet

If you have any known food allergies, sensitivities, or intolerances, remove the offending foods right away. Also remove the most common allergens, which include dairy, gluten, soy, sugar, yeast, and alcohol, from your diet. Stick to a diet that is rich in vegetables, high-quality meats, and healthy fats.

Testing for Infections

If you suspect a yeast overgrowth or bacterial infection, you'll need the help of a naturopath or functional medicine doctor to diagnose it. You may need to undergo stool testing to test for bacteria or parasites or blood or urine testing to test for the presence of *Candida*. You can also request a breath test for SIBO. Work with your doctor to determine which tests are right for you.

FACT

A functional medicine doctor address the underlying causes of symptoms and disease and uses a whole-body approach to correcting the physiological imbalance causing those symptoms. A naturopathic doctor is educated in both traditional and holistic approaches to treatment of disease.

Replace

The replace portion of the program is all about adding back the nutrients and other things you need, like enzymes, for a healthy gut. These things help heal the gut and protect it from further damage. They are essential for proper digestion and absorption. There are a number of supplements available for digestive support, but working with a functional medicine doctor is the best way to find out which supplements are right for you and your level of gut health.

Reinoculate

When it comes to restoring your gut's integrity, removing the bad is only half the battle; you must also replace the good. Leaky gut takes a toll on the good bacteria in your gut. When the balance of good bacteria is off, they are unable to protect your body like they should and it can lead to sickness and disease. Probiotics help reinoculate, or repopulate, the intestines with the proper bacteria that they need to thrive.

Repair

Once you've removed toxic substances and replaced the missing beneficial bacteria in your gut, you have to give your body the tools it needs to repair its intestinal lining. Some supplements that may help the gut repair itself include glutamine, methionine, N-acetyl cysteine, and zinc. Work with your functional medicine doctor to develop the best supplement regimen to help you repair your gut.

Keep in mind that the process doesn't happen overnight. It requires patience, diligence, and commitment. Since everyone is different, there's no way to say how long you'll need to stay on a gut-healing protocol. The best thing to do is work with a naturopath or functional medicine doctor who can help recommend the proper changes and monitor your progress.

Recommended Supplements

While some supplements may help support gut health, randomly taking supplements with no real direction can be counterproductive. If you don't know if you need a certain supplement, don't just take it because it's good for your gut in theory. Work with a professional who can give you the proper tests to make the right supplement recommendations.

ALERT

Although many supplements are natural, they can still do harm to your body if not taken carefully and in the recommended dosages. Work with your functional medicine doctor to figure out which gut supplements are right for you and how much of a specific supplement you need to take.

It may take some experimentation and trial and error, but eventually you'll find the regimen that your body needs.

Probiotics

Leaky gut is most often accompanied by an imbalance in the good, or friendly, bacteria that live in your gut. These bacteria don't just help you break down and digest your food, they also play a role in your immune system and help prevent the overgrowth of bad bacteria. When good bacteria are destroyed from poor diet, antibiotic use, or chronic inflammation, they can no longer do their job, a job that is extremely important to your overall gut health.

Taking a probiotic can help restore the balance of good bacteria in your gut so that your intestines are able to repair. Not all probiotic supplements are created equal. Choose one that contains 25–100 billion units per capsule and at least five different bacterial strains. Some of the most potent strains are *L. acidophilus* or *B. bifidum*, so look for one that contains these as well as a combination of others. Keep in mind that probiotics contain live organisms that cannot survive in hot temperatures. As a general rule, refrigerated probiotics tend to be more potent. Including fermented foods, like sauerkraut, kombucha, kimchi, kefir, and pickles can also help.

Glutamine or L-glutamine

Glutamine, also called L-glutamine, is an amino acid with the ability to repair damaged soft tissue, like that found in the inside of your intestines. The amino acid also promotes the regrowth of new gut lining and may even help reduce sugar cravings. Homemade bone broths contain glutamine, which can also be found in over-the-counter supplements.

Digestive Enzymes

Digestive enzymes assist in the breakdown and absorption of nutrients. If your body is lacking sufficient amounts of enzymes to support proper digestion, you won't be able to absorb the right amount of nutrients no matter how nutrient-dense your diet is. Enzymes work in conjunction with betaine HCl, which helps activate some of them.

Betaine HCl

Betaine HCl increases the amount of acid in your stomach, which aids the digestion of protein. The presence of adequate amounts of stomach acid also ensures that you're able to properly absorb important nutrients, like vitamin B_{12}, iron, and zinc.

Deglycyrrhizinated Licorice, or DGL

Certain components of licorice help support the lining in your stomach and your small intestine and help reduce the levels of the stress hormone cortisol in your body. Unfortunately, licorice contains a compound called glycyrrhizin that has been shown to raise blood pressure. DGL is a supplement that's been extracted from licorice root and gone through a manufacturing process that removes the glycyrrhizin so that you can reap the benefits without the drawbacks.

Other Supplements

When your body is in a state of chronic stress, as is the case with leaky gut, it depletes the minerals magnesium and zinc fairly quickly. Magnesium is important for relaxation, while zinc plays a major role in tissue repair.

ALERT

Magnesium is often used as an aid for constipation because the magnesium salts have a laxative effect. If you're taking magnesium for the first time, start with a small dose and increase gradually. The types of magnesium most likely to cause a laxative effect are magnesium carbonate, magnesium chloride, magnesium gluconate, and magnesium oxide.

Work with your functional medicine doctor or naturopath to find the right doses of supplements that are right for you.

CHAPTER 5

Changing Your Diet to Support Gut Health

Everyone is unique; that's what makes this world an interesting place. That's also why there's no perfect, one-size-fits-all diet for supporting gut health. Your ideal diet may look completely different from the one that works best for your mom or brother or neighbor or coworker. Your body knows what it wants and it knows what it doesn't and it's usually not shy about telling you. You just have to listen.

Following an Elimination Diet

The first step to restoring your gut health is to clear your gut of any toxins and identify the foods that are harmful to you. Certain foods should be eliminated by everyone; others might be a problem for you specifically, but may be perfectly fine for other people. To reach your own optimal health, you must identify and eliminate the foods that you're sensitive to.

What to Avoid

Elimination diets are free from any foods that are known to contribute to gut dysfunction. These foods include:

- Gluten
- Non-gluten grains (including corn)
- Dairy
- Soy
- Refined sugars
- Nuts
- Beans and legumes
- Citrus fruit
- Alcohol
- Caffeine

Remove all of these gut-damaging foods from your diet for a minimum of 30 days. Prior to starting your elimination diet, it's a good idea to begin a food journal. In this journal, record what you eat and any symptoms you experience, whether or not you think they're related to the food you're eating. Remember, symptoms may be common, but they're not normal.

ESSENTIAL

Don't get caught up in trying to track calories or how many carbohydrates you're eating. This is not the focus of an elimination diet. The purpose of the elimination diet is to identify any foods that may be causing damage to your gut.

Once you start your elimination diet, continue to track your food and any symptoms. Note if any symptoms are improving or even disappearing. If you're still experiencing symptoms or any symptoms are getting worse, note that too.

At the end of the 30 days, you will go through a reintroduction period. This reintroduction period will allow you to determine which foods are safe to bring back into your diet and which foods you should ditch for good. While you may be able to tolerate some foods like non-gluten grains and dairy occasionally, it's advantageous to remove gut-damaging foods like gluten, refined sugar, soy, and processed foods from your diet permanently.

Reintroduction

The point of the elimination diet is not so much removing the foods as reintroducing them. Doing a proper reintroduction is the only way to isolate foods that may be causing any symptoms. After 30 days on the elimination diet, reintroduce foods one at a time and monitor yourself for symptoms. For example, if you decide to reintroduce dairy, have some butter with breakfast, a piece of cheese at lunch, and a glass of milk with dinner. On the next day, go back to your elimination diet, removing dairy once again, and keep track of any symptoms you experience for the next 2 days. Digestive symptoms like bloating, gas, and diarrhea are not the only clue to food sensitivities. Note changes in mood and energy levels. Pay attention to any skin trouble, like itching or hives.

ESSENTIAL

Take your time with the reintroduction phase. Finding out which foods make you feel less-than-ideal is the whole point of doing the elimination diet. If you rush through reintroduction or you reintroduce several food groups at a time, you may not be able to isolate potential food triggers and you'll have to start all over.

After 2 days and after any symptoms have gone away, reintroduce the next food. Even if you don't have any symptoms from dairy, go back to the elimination diet before reintroducing the next food item. If you choose nuts, have some walnuts with breakfast, some almond butter at lunch, and some pistachios after dinner. Note any symptoms or reactions. Keep going with this process until you've gone through the reintroduction process for all of the foods you eliminated during your elimination diet. If you found that certain foods, like nuts and dairy, don't cause you any distress, it's now safe to add them back into your diet. If you had a reaction to anything, like gluten, it's best to avoid it completely going forward.

A Natural, Real-Foods Approach

During your elimination diet and after, focus on filling your plate with natural, real foods. Vegetables should take up about 80 percent of your plate, while high-quality proteins and fat make up the remaining 20 percent. Fruits are full of beneficial nutrients, but should not take up a significant percentage of your plate. You can add a piece of fruit to your balanced meal or snack on one to two pieces of fruit throughout the day.

You don't have to measure out foods, just eyeball it and do your best to stick to this ratio. It's also important to focus on the quality of the food you eat. The better the quality, the better for your body.

Food Quality

Purchase organic fruit and vegetables that are free of chemicals and pesticides. While getting organic produce from your grocery store is good, local farmers' markets are better. Get to know farmers in your area and ask them questions about how they grow their produce. Many local farmers can't afford to get the official organic label through the government, but they still use organic growing practices.

Eat with the seasons. If a fruit or vegetable doesn't grow in the winter where you live, skip it at the grocery store until spring or summer, the time it naturally grows. Your body was meant to eat with the seasons. This helps prevent food sensitivities and ensures that you're getting a wide range of nutrients from foods that you may not normally eat.

In his book *In Defense of Food: An Eater's Manifesto*, Michael Pollan states, "You are what what you eat eats too." Keep this in mind when choosing which meat you purchase. Many conventional meats come from cows, pigs, and chickens that are fed a grain- or corn-rich diet. Conventional farmers give grain and corn to animals in an attempt to fatten them up quickly and inexpensively. Since this isn't the animal's natural food source, it affects the quality of the meat.

ESSENTIAL

If you can't afford to purchase all organic produce or you don't have easy access to organic foods, use the Environmental Working Group's Dirty Dozen Plus and Clean Fifteen lists to decide what you should purchase organic. The Dirty Dozen Plus list includes the produce items that contain the highest amount of pesticides, while the Clean Fifteen includes the fruit and vegetables that contain the least amount of pesticides.

The best meat carries three labels: organic, grass-fed, and pasture-raised. Do your best to choose the highest quality meats while staying within your budget. Talk to local farmers and butchers about buying meat in bulk. Often, farmers will offer a half or whole cow for purchase at a lower price per pound than if you were to buy cuts individually.

Choose eggs that are organic, free-range, and pasture-raised. These high-quality eggs contain more omega-3 fatty acids than their conventional counterparts and are often higher in vitamins A and E. This is because pasture-raised chickens eat their natural diet—grass and bugs—instead of the conventional diet of grains and corn. You can find pasture-raised eggs at some supermarkets, but do your best to find local farms that raise their own chickens and sell their eggs. You'll not only be supporting local farming, but you may also even get to know the chickens laying your eggs.

If you've reintroduced dairy and found that it doesn't affect you negatively, be choosy with your dairy sources as well. Opt for butter, cheese, and milk from grass-fed, pasture-raised cows.

Soaking Foods

Some foods are difficult for many people to digest. You can make these foods easier on your gut by soaking them before you eat them. Even if you've gone through the elimination diet and reintroduction phase and discovered that grains don't cause you any distress, consider soaking them overnight before you eat them to make it easier on your gut.

FACT

While it's best to permanently stay away from gluten-containing grains for optimal gut health, soaking non-gluten grains like quinoa, rice, and buckwheat overnight before you eat them makes them easier to digest. The same rule applies to beans, peas, and lentils.

Nuts are a good source of healthy protein and fat, but like grains and legumes, they are also difficult for some people to digest. If you've reintroduced nuts and experienced digestive problems like bloating and gas, try soaking them for a few hours before eating. This might eliminate the problem. Choose raw nuts that are unsalted, unsweetened, and don't contain any preservatives.

Try to include a healthy source of fat at every meal. While nuts are a good choice occasionally, they should not be your only fat source. Nuts are higher in omega-6 fatty acids than omega-3 fatty acids. Eating too many omega-6 fatty acids without balancing them out with omega-3 fatty acids can actually contribute to inflammation and gut damage. Vary your fat sources by including avocados, olives, olive oil, coconut oil, coconut flakes, full-fat canned coconut milk, grass-fed ghee, and grass-fed butter into your diet.

Eating Right

Eating right for your gut is not just about what you eat, but how you eat as well. Digestion is a complicated process that requires many different chemical reactions to take place at the same time. Different types of food require different enzymes and pH levels for proper breakdown. Your digestive system is designed to handle all of these chemical reactions, but when you bombard your body with a bunch of different types of foods, it can make the process more difficult. Ease your digestive burden by eating protein with vegetables instead of non-gluten grains, rice, or legumes. When eating grains, rice, or legumes, pair them with vegetables.

Timing your meals is also an important aspect of an ideal gut health diet. Again, there is no one-size-fits-all approach to how much you should eat and when, but develop a schedule that works for you and do your best to follow it. Try to eat breakfast within an hour of waking up. You may choose to eat another four small meals throughout the course of the day or eat a bigger lunch and dinner instead. Experiment with both eating plans and figure out which one makes you feel better.

Focusing on Fiber

Because grains have become such a staple in the American diet, many people fall short on fiber intake when eliminating grains from their diet. This can lead to issues with constipation, which is a real problem when trying to eliminate toxins from your body. If you've decided that grains don't work for you, focus on getting enough fiber elsewhere. Grain-free foods that are high in fiber include:

- Apples
- Raspberries
- Pears
- Split peas
- Lentils
- Beans
- Artichokes
- Green peas
- Broccoli
- Turnip greens
- Brussels sprouts

Try to include a fiber-rich food at each meal, but increase your intake gradually. If you increase the amount of fiber you eat too quickly, it can cause uncomfortable digestive symptoms. When increasing your fiber intake, increase your water intake as well. Fiber works best when it has access to plenty of water. The fiber absorbs the water, adding bulk to your stools and making them softer and easier to pass.

Avoiding Chemicals and Processed Foods

The typical modern diet is all about convenience. When it comes to food choices, the top three criteria for many people are convenience, portability, and taste. Sure, that frozen pizza may resemble pizza, but is it real? Not even close. Processed foods contain so many artificial ingredients and chemicals that your body doesn't even recognize them as food. When you regularly eat foods like this, your body responds by attacking the ingredients it doesn't recognize. The end result? A damaged gut.

ESSENTIAL

Don't be fooled by buzz phrases like *all-natural*, *gluten-free*, or *made with natural ingredients*. These phrases are designed by manufacturers to make you think a packaged food is a healthy choice even when it's not. Just because a processed food doesn't contain any gluten doesn't make it healthy; it may be filled with other gut-damaging ingredients like soy and sugar.

Make your meals at home whenever possible using fresh, whole ingredients. If portability and convenience are your concerns, spend a few hours on a day that you have some time prepping and preparing meals for the week. Cook in bulk and separate food into single-serving containers. Cut up fruit and vegetables and put them in baggies that are easy to grab on the go. Buy raw nuts and unsweetened dried fruit in bulk and put single servings into sandwich bags. Keep these bags on hand wherever you think hunger might strike unexpectedly. Put some in your desk drawer at work, leave some in the car, or keep them in your purse.

Restaurants and Eating Out

Eating out can be one of the most challenging aspects of sticking to your diet because restaurants often use inexpensive and easily accessible ingredients that aren't part of your plan. They may also use potentially harmful ingredients like MSG to increase the flavor of the food, even if it sacrifices its quality. While eating out is certainly not impossible, it does take some detective work and, often, a lot of questions. Don't be afraid to speak up and ask for what you want. Many restaurants, especially those with a well-trained chef, are more than willing to accommodate specific food requests.

Do Your Research

Always do your research before you even get to the restaurant. If you're in charge of picking the place, you can search local restaurants that have a gluten-free menu or many specialty items available. If you're lucky, you may even be able to find a farm-to-table restaurant that uses locally sourced meats and vegetables as much as possible. If you don't have the privilege of choosing where you'll eat, look up the restaurant menu online before you go. This way, you can identify your best options before you even step foot in the door.

Call Ahead

If you've looked over a restaurant's menu online and there's nothing you can or want to eat directly off the menu, call the restaurant and ask to speak to the manager. Inform the manager that you take your health very seriously and that you have some special requests. Ask the manager if the restaurant is able to accommodate them. In many cases, this won't be a problem. If it is, ask the manager if it's okay for you to bring your own meal. You may feel silly doing this at first, but your gut will thank you for it. If the manager is unwilling to accommodate any of your requests, consider choosing another location.

Inform Your Server

Even if you've done your due diligence and determined what you want to eat before you get to the restaurant, it's important to inform your server of your dietary needs just to make sure everything goes according to plan. Let your server know what foods you cannot eat and make sure that these foods are not included in your meal. Be specific and don't be afraid to ask questions. While your server may be aware that gluten is in a hamburger bun, she may not know that it's also in the flour some restaurants use to thicken sauces. Ask her if there's flour on the meat or in any sauces. Ask if the restaurant puts butter or MSG on their vegetables. If you think fresh rolls on the table will be too much of a temptation, ask to skip the bread basket.

Go Prepared

In most restaurants, you'll be able to order a piece of meat and a side of vegetables. It's the sauces and dressings that may contain ingredients that affect your gut health. Consider bringing your own salad dressing in a small container or a small shaker of your favorite vegetable seasoning. Ask for meat seasoned with only salt and pepper, plain steamed vegetables, and an undressed side salad. Toss your salad in the dressing you brought and coat your vegetables with your seasoning. It may seem like a lot of work, but it's really all about planning ahead. Eventually, it all becomes second nature.

Eating Mindfully

A meal should be something that you savor, not something that you rush through at your desk while working or in your car between errands. Part of optimal gut health is eating slowly and mindfully and enjoying every bite. When it's time to eat, stop everything else and sit down for a proper meal. Prepare your body for digestion by taking a deep breath and transitioning into a relaxed state.

FACT

Research shows that those who eat in front of the television miss cues from their body telling them that they are full and tend to eat more than they would if they were paying attention to their meal.

Put your food on a plate and sit at your kitchen or dining-room table. If you're at work, sit down in the break room. Avoid all distractions like your phone and the television. Chew each bite thoroughly and adequately. Don't just chew a piece of meat a couple times and then choke it down. Make each meal a process. You don't need to sit down for hours. The point is to pay attention to what you're doing and make mealtime all about eating.

A Sample Menu for Optimal Gut Health

Following a gut-health diet may have a learning curve, but you don't need to make it complicated. Don't get caught up in trying to prepare lavish, gourmet meals every day. Use what you have and keep it simple. A typical day may look something like this:

You wake up in the morning and start your day by drinking 2 (8-ounce) glasses of filtered water. Once your thirst is quenched and you've rubbed the sleep from your eyes, it's time for breakfast. You make a quick scrambled eggs dish by sautéing some mild-tasting veggies like onions, zucchini, and chopped spinach in coconut oil, then adding in a few whisked eggs. Once the eggs have cooked, which only takes a few minutes, you top the meal with a few slices of avocado.

ESSENTIAL

Don't be afraid of fat. Healthy fats help keep you full, allow you to absorb vital nutrients, and lubricate the digestive system. Try to include a good source of fat, such as avocado, coconut oil, or coconut flakes, at every meal.

You drink some more water from your water bottle on your way to work. A few hours later you start to feel hungry again, so you pull out a snack: an apple you sliced last night. You top it with the almond butter you keep stashed in your desk drawer. When it's time for lunch, you sit down in the break room and take out the salad you prepared: mixed greens, cucumbers, red onion, a handful of walnuts, a hard-boiled egg, some slices of avocado, and canned tuna topped with olive oil, lemon juice, and a shake or two of pepper.

Once late afternoon rolls around, you start to feel like you could use a snack to get you through until dinnertime, so you open your drawer and pull out one of the snacks you keep in there: a sandwich bag with a serving of nuts, dried fruit, and unsweetened coconut flakes. You drink more water while you finish the day's work.

You're tired when you get home so you want a quick dinner. You season a couple of chicken thighs with salt, pepper, and paprika and put them in a hot pan coated in coconut oil. While the chicken cooks, you wash some broccoli and put it in a steaming pot to cook. When it's done, you toss the broccoli in extra-virgin olive oil and top it with some pepper and chunky sea salt.

Of course, your day won't look exactly like this, but it's a basic template when eating for gut health. Focus on real, whole foods, cook them yourself whenever possible, and always be prepared. It's important to remember that complete change doesn't happen overnight. It's unrealistic to think that you're going to go from a processed-food-laden diet to a perfectly clean gut-health diet overnight. Make small changes every day and do the best you can until you reach your goals. Your gut, and the rest of your body, will thank you.

CHAPTER 6

Balancing Bacteria in Your Gut

Your gut is home to 100 trillion bacteria or about 2–3 pounds' worth. It may be unnerving to know that you have 3 pounds of bacteria lining your intestinal tract, but when you consider the wide variety of roles these bacteria play in keeping you healthy, you might just start to consider them your best friends. The bacteria in your gut help promote normal digestive function, but they also comprise more than 75 percent of your immune system. In short: if your gut isn't healthy, then the rest of you won't be healthy. Good bugs, good bacteria, healthy gut flora: it doesn't matter what you call them, the bacteria in your gut help you thrive.

Good and Bad Gut Bacteria

The population of bacteria in your gut is a combination of both good and "bad" bacteria, but before you start worrying about the bad bacteria, keep in mind that the bacteria isn't inherently bad, per se. It becomes problematic when the numbers get out of control. The key to maintaining good health is to keep a healthy balance of both good and bad bacteria in your gut.

Good Bugs

There are so many bacteria living in your gut that scientists have not been able to identify all of them. They do estimate that there are between 300 and 1,000 different species. Of these, 30–40 strains account for about 90 percent of the bacterial population and do most of the work in your gut. Many of these species fall under the *Bifidobacterium* and *Lactobacillus* genera.

Bifidobacterium

Scientists have identified about 32 different species of *Bifidobacteria* to date. Most *Bifidobacteria*, which are similar in genetic makeup, are found in the large intestine—more specifically, the colon. Like other strains of bacteria, *Bifidobacteria* produce vitamins, antibacterial chemicals, and lactic acid; however, a unique feature of *Bifidobacteria* is that they also produce acetic acid, which helps fight off the growth of potentially harmful bacteria, like *E. coli*, and yeast, like *Candida*. Your body can also use acetic acid as a source of energy. *Bifidobacteria* also help break down any proteins that reach the colon without being fully digested in the stomach and small intestine so that they do not rot in the large intestine. Some species of *Bifidobacteria* include *B. longum*, *B. lactis*, and *B. bifidum*.

FACT

Acetic acid is more effective at preventing the overgrowth of yeast and mold than lactic acid, which is a byproduct of most of the bacteria that live in the gut. Because of this, large amounts of *Bifidobacteria* are found in the colon, where slow fecal transmit time makes disease more likely.

Lactobacillus

The *Lactobacillus* genus is arguably the most well-known strain of good bacteria, encompassing about 25 different species of bacteria. Like *Bifido-bacteria*, *Lactobacillus* produces lactic acid, which helps maintain the intestinal barrier, prevents infection, and acts as an anti-inflammatory agent. *Lactobacillus* also helps promote mucus production in the small intestine. Adequate mucus production ensures that things flow through the intestine smoothly. Some species of *Lactobacillus* include *L. casei*, *L. acidophilus*, and *L. bulgaricus*.

Bad Bugs

Bacteria only become problematic or "bad" when their numbers get so large that the good bacteria can no longer control them. You can live perfectly healthily with some potentially disease-causing bacteria in your system, but when their population grows, health problems and disease are more likely. Some bacteria strains that have the potential to cause disease include *Salmonella* and *Clostridium*. Luckily, the number of good bacteria far outweighs the bad. If you keep your gut flora intact, you can protect yourself from problems.

Salmonella

When your gut is inflamed, it gives potentially harmful bacteria like *Salmonella*, which can cause food poisoning, a fighting chance. Research shows that inflammation makes it easier for *Salmonella* to invade the intestinal lining and survive there.

Clostridium

Clostridium bacteria normally live in your gut in perfect harmony with the rest of the gut flora. When the numbers of good bacteria are diminished, *Clostridium*, specifically *C. difficile*, has a chance to thrive. When numbers of *C. difficile* grow, they produce toxins that attack your intestinal wall and cause uncomfortable symptoms.

E. coli

E. coli, or *Escherichia coli,* has gotten such a bad rap that it may be hard to believe that this bacterial strain actually lives happily in your gut under normal circumstances. When numbers of *E. coli* are allowed to grow, however, the bacteria can overtake other bacterial strains, damage the gut, and contribute to chronic diarrhea and inflammatory bowel disease, or IBD. *E. coli* use a byproduct of inflammation—called nitrate—to produce energy and grow.

QUESTION

Am I at risk for a *C. difficile* infection?
The risk for developing a *C. difficile* infection increases with antibiotic exposure, use of proton pump inhibitors, decreased immunity, and gastrointestinal surgery. A lengthy stay in a hospital setting or a serious underlying illness can also increase your risk of developing an infection. Initial symptoms of a *C. difficile* infection include diarrhea and stomach cramps. As the infection progresses, it can lead to fever, nausea, vomiting, weakness, dehydration, and blood in the stool.

Small Intestinal Bacterial Overgrowth

Your small intestine normally contains low levels of bacteria. The bulk of the bacterial population is found in the large intestine, where they help finish up the process of digestion. In the case of small intestinal bacterial overgrowth, or SIBO, bacteria from the large intestine invade the upper area of the small intestine, where a large portion of digestion takes place. When the bacteria in the small intestine reach high numbers—more than 100,000 per millimeter in the case of SIBO—they produce enzymes, toxins, and gases like carbon dioxide and methane. These bacterial byproducts don't just cause digestive distress, they also interfere with normal digestion. If left to their own devices, the bacteria can eventually damage the lining of the small intestine.

When that happens, it can lead to chronic health problems including:

- Irritable bowel syndrome
- Diverticulosis
- Fibromyalgia
- Celiac disease
- Crohn's disease
- Autoimmune diseases
- Chronic acid reflux

The best way to reduce the numbers of potentially harmful bacteria is to starve them of their food source. Bacteria feed off carbohydrates, specifically hard-to-digest carbohydrates like fructose (fruit sugar), lactose (milk sugar), starch, fiber, and sugar alcohols, like xylitol and sorbitol. Cutting these carbohydrates out of your diet may have a beneficial effect on bacterial overgrowth.

Healthy Gut Flora

Having a healthy balance of bacteria in your gut aids in digestion, including the absorption of nutrients and the formation of stool, and supports your immune function. Having a diverse population of bacteria in your gut also helps your body use insulin effectively, reducing your risk of metabolic diseases, like diabetes. Because this gut flora is so vital to your overall health, it's important to restore or maintain the balance of these microorganisms.

Gut Flora and Digestion

Perhaps the best-known function of the bacteria in your gut is their role in digestion. The different species of bacteria in your gut have different DNA patterns. These DNA patterns determine what they do. Some bacteria are coded to digest carbohydrates and sugars, while others digest protein or fat. For optimal digestion, it's important to have a balance of the bacteria that perform different digestive functions. If your body cannot digest and absorb nutrients properly, it can lead to nutritional deficiencies and a host of uncomfortable symptoms—like fatigue, anemia, and low energy—that come with them.

Good bacteria also break down certain carbohydrates like resistant starches, cellulose, and pectins that you wouldn't be able to digest without them. The bacteria turn these carbohydrates into short-chain fatty acids, which your body can use as energy. Short-chain fatty acids also help with the repair of damaged intestinal cells and the growth of new ones.

FACT

When you don't have a good balance of different types of bacteria in your gut, partially digested material remains stagnant and starts to go rancid. This leads to digestive symptoms like belching, bloating, abdominal pain, and increased flatulence.

Some bacteria produce vitamins, like vitamin K and the B vitamins folate, B_{12}, and biotin, and others improve the absorption of minerals, like copper, iron, magnesium, and manganese. Good bacteria also help promote proper elimination and prevent digestive symptoms like bloating and gas.

Gut Flora and Immune Function

Your immune system consists of physical structures and innate and adaptive processes that protect your body. The physical part of your immune system includes your hair, skin, tears, saliva, and mucous membranes. These structures literally form a physical barrier between you and the outside world. Your body does its best to keep potentially harmful organisms out by using its physical immune system.

Your innate immune system is your body's automatic response to foreign invaders. If bacteria or viruses make it past your physical immune system, your body instinctively knows what to do. It sends out antibodies to attack potentially harmful organisms and sets the wheels of inflammation in motion to protect open wounds.

The adaptive immune system is one that your body learns over time. When you're exposed to a certain bacterium or virus repeatedly, your body will eventually learn how to respond to that organism properly.

Your gut flora plays a role in each area of your immune system. It forms a physical barrier by lining the inside of your intestines and literally preventing potentially harmful bacteria from camping out and growing there or making its way into the blood through the intestinal wall. This is known as the barrier effect or colonization resistance. When there are a large number of healthy bacteria, they are also able to eat up all the food and prevent the bad bugs from getting any, effectively starving them out. The good bugs in your digestive tract also have an ability to communicate with your immune system.

When an organism with the potential to cause sickness makes its way through the digestive tract, the good bacteria can send a message to your immune system to attack and destroy it before it has a chance to cause illness. Some bacteria in your gut also have an ability to produce antibiotic and antifungal agents, which fight infection on their own.

Use of antibiotics disrupts the balance of your gut flora. Broad-spectrum antibiotics don't discriminate between the good and the bad. In fact, the good bacteria are more susceptible to them than the bad. While antibiotics have been a vital part of human survival over the years, problems arise with overuse, overprescribing, and neglecting to repopulate the good bacteria once the course of antibiotics has ended.

Gut Flora and Stress

An imbalance in your gut flora doesn't just affect you physically, it can affect you mentally. Studies show that having an overgrowth of certain bacteria, like *C. difficle*, in the gut can trigger a systemic stress response that keeps you in fight or flight mode, which is characterized by increased heart rate, high blood pressure, increased blood glucose, difficulty focusing, and slowed digestion, at all times. Staying in fight or flight long-term can cause chronic inflammation that leads to chronic diseases. Conversely, having the "right" balance of *Bifidobacterium* and *Lactobacillus* can turn off the hormonal signals that cause that chronic stress response.

Importance of Probiotics

Probiotics are live cultures that provide some type of benefit to the host—you. In the case of gut dysbiosis, probiotics help repopulate the gut with good bacteria to help restore the balance. There are two major ways to introduce probiotics into your gut.

Fermented Foods

Fermented foods are not a new thing; in fact, fermented foods have fallen out of fashion with a rise in the processing, pasteurization, and preservation of modern society. Fermented foods are those that have been preserved using a process called lacto-fermentation. During this process, bacteria feed on the sugars and starches naturally present in the food.

ESSENTIAL

Fermentation does more than increase a food's shelf life. It makes the food more digestible, changes flavor and texture, reduces the presence of carbohydrates known for causing gas, and synthesizes vitamins, like vitamin B_{12}.

This process not only preserves the food, it creates enzymes, fatty acids, and various strains of probiotics. You can help repopulate your gut with beneficial bacteria by making fermented foods a part of your daily diet. Some examples of fermented foods include yogurt, kimchi, sauerkraut, and pickles. You can also consume probiotics by drinking fermented beverages like kombucha and kefir.

Supplements

If your gut is really lacking in healthy bacteria, diet alone may not be enough to bring your numbers back up to normal. Remember, a healthy gut contains trillions of bacteria and sometimes yogurt and sauerkraut just aren't enough to get you where you need to be. In these cases, taking a high-dose probiotic regularly is important. With the rising focus on gut health also came a rise in available probiotic supplements. It's important that you know what to look for when choosing a probiotic supplement because they are not all created equal.

Choosing the Right Supplement

One probiotic capsule can contain anywhere from 1 billion to 100 billion (or even more) bacteria. Generally, the more potent an individual capsule is, the better; however, when taking probiotics for the first time, it may be beneficial to start with smaller doses to avoid a severe die-off reaction. Start with a probiotic that contains 50 billion bacteria per capsule and work your way up, if necessary.

ESSENTIAL

A die-off reaction happens when pathogens—like the bad bacteria in your gut—give off toxins as they die. A die-off reaction may cause fever, chills, headaches, skin rashes, brain fog, digestive distress, muscle aches, and increased mucus production. These reactions typically last less than a week, but if you experience severe symptoms, you may want to scale back on your probiotic dose.

Some probiotics contain only one strain of bacteria, while others contain more than two dozen. Since you can't pinpoint which strain or strains of bacteria your gut is low in, it's best to choose a capsule that contains at least a few different strains. Choose one that contains a few of the most potent strains, such as *L. acidophilus* or *B. bifidum*, as well as a combination of others.

Probiotics are living organisms, so proper storage is vital. Pay attention to storage instructions, no matter what type of probiotic you choose. Many probiotics require refrigeration and those that don't often need to be kept in a cool place. If probiotics aren't stored correctly, they'll eventually die, making them useless. Keep in mind that probiotics also have an expiration date. It's best to buy in smaller quantities so that you don't have a lot of capsules sitting around approaching or passing their expiration date.

You should start to notice a difference in how you feel after a couple weeks of taking probiotics. If you don't notice any changes, consider increasing your dose or trying a probiotic with a different combination of bacterial strains. Because it's impossible to determine which strain or strains of bacteria your body is low in, it can take some trial and error before you find a probiotic that works for you.

ALERT

Always buy probiotics from a reputable source. A good place to start is your local health food store, your naturopath or functional medicine doctor, or directly from a well-known manufacturer. Some probiotics that are sold online through unknown sources are fake. At best, these probiotics contain useless ingredients that won't improve your health; at worst, they contain dangerous ingredients that may do damage to your body.

Fixing Bacterial Imbalance

Correcting bacterial imbalance requires a multifaceted approach. There is no miracle or quick fix; it requires several changes in diet and lifestyle habits. The amount of time it takes to bring the bacteria in your gut back to a healthy balance depends on several factors, including the amount of damage to your gut flora and your willingness to adhere to a lifestyle that allows good bacteria to thrive.

Diet

Keep in mind that every time you take a bite, you're not only feeding yourself, you're also either feeding or starving the bacteria in your gut. An essential first step to correcting bacterial imbalance is to change your diet. Avoid sugar, refined grains, and processed foods, which provide a food source for the bad bacteria in your gut. Consume plenty of fermented foods or a probiotic supplement every day. Eat plenty of fermentable fibers, like sweet potatoes, yams, and yucca, which help feed the good bugs.

Stress Management

Chronic stress alters the function of your immune system. This results in an increase in inflammatory agents in the blood and a decrease in beneficial bacteria. If you experience chronic stress or feel anxious all the time, figure out a way to manage this stress in a healthy way. Take yoga classes, learn to meditate, or start a journal. Talk to a professional who can help you manage disruptive thinking patterns. Take a little time each day to do something fun or engage in an activity that allows you to be creative, such as writing, drawing, or making a collage.

Avoidance of Medication

Antibiotics, anti-inflammatory medications, like aspirin and ibuprofen, and acid blockers, like antacids, cause damage to the intestinal lining and kill off good bacteria. Avoid the use of these medications when trying to restore a healthy gut balance. If you're currently on a prescription medication and want to discontinue use, talk to your doctor about the proper way to wean yourself off it.

Taking It a Step Further

Restoring healthy gut flora doesn't happen overnight; have patience and trust the process. If you're following these steps and still not seeing any difference within a few weeks, you may have an underlying infection, such as a parasite or *Candida* overgrowth. You can request specialized testing like stool testing or organic acid testing from your functional medicine doctor to determine if there's an underlying issue hindering your success. If there is, your doctor can put you on a strict diet and supplement regimen that will help rid your body of the infection so that you can work to restore gut function.

CHAPTER 7

Hydration and Exercise

When it comes to gut health, diet and proper supplementation are only half of the battle. Eating real, whole foods and taking the supplements that will help get your gut back in balance put you on the right track, but drinking clean water and getting regular exercise are two other factors that are critical to reaching your optimal health.

Water, Your Body, and Your Gut

Your body's need for water comes second only to its need for oxygen. You could live for several weeks without food but would only survive a few days without water. That's because your body relies on water to carry out almost every physiological process necessary for survival.

The average adult is made up of about 60 percent water, although the exact amount varies depending on several factors, including age, gender, and muscle tone. Muscle tissue is comprised of about 65 percent water, while fat tissue clocks in at 10–40 percent.

General Functions of Water

Water is often referred to as the universal solvent because most substances dissolve in it. This characteristic of water is important because it's what allows the chemical reactions in your body to take place. When certain compounds come into contact with water, they break down into individual molecules. When certain molecules meet, chemical reactions, like the ones that provide you with the energy you need to survive, take place.

FACT

So many substances are able to dissolve in water because of its polarity. The hydrogen side of each water molecule carries a slight positive charge, while the oxygen side carries a slight negative charge. This helps water pull the compounds apart, allowing their ions to form new compounds.

Water also transports waste products and toxins from the body, acts as a lubricant and cushion around joints, serves as a shock absorber inside the eyes and spinal cord, aids in the body's temperature regulation, and helps maintain blood volume.

Water and Your Gut

Healthy digestion requires that you're well hydrated. The enzymes in your saliva must dissolve in water, which makes up the bulk of saliva, in order to start the breakdown of starches in your mouth. You also need water to digest soluble fiber. Without adequate amounts of water, you run the risk of becoming constipated.

If you're not drinking enough, your colon steals water from the waste material and pulls it back into the body. This results in water-deprived stools that are small and hard. These hard, dry stools are difficult to pass because they stick to the dry wall of the colon. By drinking plenty of water each day, you help your body stay hydrated, so it doesn't need to extract much water from the solid waste materials that are moving through the colon. Since the waste material keeps its water, it stays soft and pliable and is able to move through the colon at a much easier and faster rate.

ESSENTIAL

Warm water with lemon is a soothing digestive tonic that can help keep you regular. Heat 8–10 ounces of water and add the juice of a lemon. For a little variation, use lime instead of lemon juice, or add a slice of fresh ginger or a mint or basil leaf.

Your gut also needs water to help move bacteria and waste through the digestive tract. When you don't drink enough water, the bacteria in your gut can become imbalanced, which leads to issues like bloating and chronic inflammation.

Water Loss

On a normal day, you can lose up to 1 quart of water just through normal body functions like perspiration, urination, and breathing. If you exercise daily, you're likely losing even more than that. When you get rid of fluid, you also dump electrolytes, which are minerals like sodium and calcium that keep your body's fluids balanced. If you exercise, mow the lawn, or forget to drink as much water as you should, your body may become dehydrated, a state in which you've lost more water than you're taking in. It's important to replace the water you lose to keep your body functioning optimally and to prevent the symptoms of dehydration.

Mild dehydration signs include:

- Thirst
- Flushed face
- Dry, warm skin
- Lightheadedness or dizziness made worse when you stand
- Weakness
- Cramping in the arms and legs
- Having few or no tears
- Headache
- A lack of energy
- Dry mouth and tongue with thick saliva

Even becoming mildly dehydrated, or losing as little as 1–2 percent of your body weight, can seriously impact your body's ability to function. It is fairly easy to become dehydrated. In fact, researchers suspect that 75 percent of Americans have mild, chronic dehydration. By the time you become thirsty, your body is telling you it's dehydrated.

How Much Do You Need?

For a long time, the general recommendation was to drink 8 (8-ounce) glasses of water per day. That isn't the best guide since everybody is different and individual needs vary. Your personal water needs are influenced by your physical activity level, your diet, and environmental factors like the temperature of the air around you. However, the new basic guideline for how much water you need is to divide your weight in half and then drink that many ounces of water each day. This means a 160-pound person needs 80 ounces, while a 200-pound person needs 100 ounces.

Timing Your Intake

When it comes to gut health, when you drink is just as important as how much you drink. Drinking beverages with meals has become the norm, but it's actually not the best practice for your gut. When you drink with your meals, it dilutes the amount of hydrochloric acid in your stomach. As you now know, hydrochloric acid is vital to activating the enzymes that allow you to properly digest protein. When HCl is diluted, it stalls protein breakdown and hinders digestion.

Cold beverages take an extra toll on digestion because when your water is ice-cold, your body uses energy that it would normally be using for digestion to bring that water up to body temperature. As a result, digestion is hindered. Drink your beverages about 30 minutes before or 30–60 minutes after your meals and skip the ice, if you can.

Choosing Your Water Source

When working to clean up your diet and clear your gut of toxins, it's important not to overlook your water source. Water is in every nook and cranny of your body: It travels to your brain, it makes up the bulk of your blood, and it lubricates your intestinal tract. If your water is contaminated or inundated with chemicals from treatment processes, it can leave toxins in every part of your body and negate all the hard work you're doing. While it's tempting to fill up a glass from your tap, doing so may be doing more harm than you realize.

Tap Water

Tap water always contains more than just water. Tap water is often contaminated with toxic heavy metals like lead or cadmium and with the remnants of prescription medications that people flush down their toilets. Tap water is also treated with fluoride and chlorine, which are meant to kill any pathogens and keep the pipes from rusting, but create a whole host of problems. Fluoride is associated with an increased risk of cancer, digestive disorders, and kidney disease. Chlorine is known to kill many of the good bacteria and other microbes that live in your intestinal tract and protect the health of your gut.

An area's water source can also become contaminated in a number of different ways. Industrial chemicals and wastes, pesticides, and other farm chemicals often seep through the soil to contaminate the water that ends up in your cup. Even though the individual chemicals are bad enough, volatile chemicals can combine with other chemicals, like chlorine, to form even more toxic products.

Well Water

Getting your water from a well has its own concerns. According to the CDC, contaminated private well water causes one-fourth of the drinking water outbreaks that make people sick. Runoff pollutants can also seep into groundwater, and microorganisms, heavy metals like lead and copper, household waste, fluoride, and more can all be found in traces in ground water. If it's in the groundwater, it's in your well.

FACT

You should have your well water tested annually, but do it sooner if there are known problems with well water in your area or you have experienced problems near your well, such as flooding or land disturbances. Test your water more frequently if there are waste disposal sites nearby or immediately after you replace or repair any part of your well system.

If you are a homeowner with a private well, you should test your well water annually to make sure you've got safe drinking water. Contact your health or environmental department, or a private laboratory to test for germs and harmful chemicals. The CDC recommends testing for fecal coliform, nitrates, volatile organic compounds, and pH levels. If you live near farm animals, heavy industrial sites, or commercial agriculture fields, you may be at a higher risk for pollutants.

Bottled Water

Bottled water's popularity is fueled in part by suspicions over the quality of tap water; but you may not be getting what you pay for. Even though the label may say pure, bottlers are required in most cases only to meet the same quality standards as tap water. A study published in the scientific journal *PLOS ONE* reported that a single bottle of water can contain upward of 24,500 different chemicals. Many of these chemicals mimic the effect of potent pharmaceutical drugs, while others were classified as endocrine-disrupting chemicals, or EDCs. EDCs can interfere with your hormonal systems and have been linked to the development of breast cancer.

Even if you are drinking real spring water, the bottle itself might make you sick. Many plastic bottles contain bisphenol A, or BPA. Low-dose exposure to BPA has been linked to cancer, diabetes, fertility problems, and behavior disorders in children.

In 2012, the FDA banned the use of BPA in baby bottles and children's cups, but it may still be present in the average water bottle. In addition, many manufacturers use a chemical named DEHF, which is used to make plastic bottles more flexible. Like EDCs, DEHF interferes with hormonal signaling. If you won't ditch the plastic for good, be smarter about it. Choose bottled waters that actually come from a spring. Don't rely on a misleading brand name. Read the labels and look for the phrase *natural spring water*. Don't reuse plastic water bottles and don't put them in the freezer. Throw out any water bottles that have been sitting in a hot car for an extended period of time. Extreme temperatures can accelerate the leaching of chemicals into the water.

Water Filtration Options

Your best bet is to drink filtered water. There are many filtration systems available and each has its own pros and cons. A common and inexpensive way to filter your water is to use a filtration pitcher or a faucet-mounted filter. These filters work in the same way: Water passes through an activated carbon filter and chlorine, mercury, and lead levels are reduced. They may also reduce the amount of chemicals that end up in the water as a byproduct of disinfection, but not as effectively as other filters. Both filtration pitchers and faucet-mounted filters require frequent filter changes.

FACT

Activated charcoal is charcoal that has been exposed to oxygen in order to open up the spaces between the carbon atoms. These tiny openings attract and absorb impurities present in your water. Activated charcoal is especially good at trapping chlorine, but may miss other impurities like sodium or nitrates.

If you want something a little more extensive, you can opt for an under-the-sink filter. These filters are fitted to the water supply by a plumber and use a variety of filtration techniques that are usually more effective than pitcher or faucet filters. Under-the-sink filters require less frequent filter changes.

The king of water filtration systems is a whole-house system that is installed right at your home's main water source. These filtration systems can be expensive, but are often a worthy investment in your health. In addition to filtering your drinking water, home filtration systems filter your shower and bath water.

Filtering your bath water is just as important as, if not more important than, filtering your drinking water. It is estimated that two-thirds of your harmful exposure to chlorine comes from the absorption of water and inhalation of steam during a shower. Taking a 10-minute shower in chlorinated water is equivalent to drinking 6–8 glasses of contaminated water. If you sit in the bath regularly, your exposure is even greater.

QUESTION

I have questions about my drinking water. Whom should I call?
A good place to start is the Environmental Protection Agency's Safe Drinking Water Hotline: 1-800-426-4791. It's free and offers information on local drinking water quality, drinking water standards, public drinking water systems, and wells.

You may want to start small with a pitcher filter and then work your way to a whole-house system when it works with your budget. Either way, take the steps to start filtering some, if not all, of your water today.

Beverages to Limit

Just because it's liquid doesn't mean it's hydrating or helpful. Plus, depending on the drink, you might be adding more risks to your digestive health. Every time you choose a glass of soda, for example, you are robbing your body of valuable nutrients. Sodas can also leach calcium from your bones and damage the enamel on your teeth. The phosphoric acid in sodas can contribute to bloating, acid reflux, and heartburn, while the sugar feeds the bad bacteria and yeast that may be present in your gut.

Beverages to limit include:

- Soda
- Alcohol
- Fruit juices
- Sweetened teas
- Artificial lemonades
- Other sugar-sweetened beverages

Alcohol damages the health of the gut, especially if you drink it on an empty stomach. In addition, the sugar in alcohol contributes to the overgrowth of yeast and bacterial imbalance. If you're looking to liven up your water, add fresh fruit chunks, some sprigs of mint, or some cucumber slices.

If you want to drink something besides water, choose unsweetened herbal teas or homemade bone broth. The collagen and gelatin in bone broth help protect and soothe the lining of the digestive tract. Collagen also helps heal your gut lining and reduces inflammation in the gut. Try to drink a cup of homemade bone broth—made using bones from pasture-raised animals—every day.

Benefits of Exercise

It should come as no surprise that exercise is good for you. Regular exercise makes you stronger and helps you feel better. It helps support the balance of microorganisms in your gut and keeps your digestive system moving. It also helps to:

- Control your weight
- Reduce physical and mental stress
- Improve digestion
- Sharpen your mental acuity and ability to concentrate
- Strengthen the cardiovascular system
- Lubricate joints
- Strengthen your heart
- Improve mineral uptake in the skeleton
- Lower your cholesterol and triglyceride levels
- Increase your circulation

Besides boosting your overall wellness, a regular fitness program can cut your risk of developing diabetes, breast and colon cancer, osteoporosis, kidney disease, high blood pressure, and arthritis.

ESSENTIAL

As a general rule, you should aim for at least 30 minutes of physical activity every day. Depending on your health and fitness goals, this may be the bare minimum. For optimal health benefits, increase your exercise to 300 minutes per week.

Exercise is also important for mental health. When you exercise, your brain releases endorphins, natural painkillers and antidepressants that help improve your mood. Exercise also helps to balance serotonin, another feel-good hormone. When you exercise you feel better, stronger, healthier, and you have more self-confidence.

Exercise and Gut Health

While most people know that exercise offers overall health benefits, many don't know that it's good for your gut health, too. A study published in the medical journal *Gut* reported that athletes had a larger diversity of microorganisms in their digestive tract than sedentary non-athletes. This is important because people with a diverse population of germs in their gut are less prone to obesity and less likely to develop immune problems and other health disorders.

These athletes also had higher numbers of a particular bacterium called *Akkermansiaceae*. High levels of *Akkermansiaceae* have been linked to less widespread inflammation and a decreased risk for obesity. The sedentary individuals in the study had less diverse populations of microbes as well as lower numbers of *Akkermansiaceae*.

Regular exercise also contributes to gut health by preventing and/or alleviating constipation. Exercise stimulates intestinal muscles to contract, which causes them to push digested material through your system. Even very gentle exercise works the muscles of the bowel, triggering peristalsis, and helps the colon to return to a pattern of normal contractions.

Exercise can help reduce the risk of colon cancer and help the body absorb nutrients more effectively. Exercise also helps gas pass through the digestive system, helping to reduce bloat and abdominal pain. Because exercise is effective in reducing stress, it can also help you with digestive symptoms related to anxiety and tension.

Types of Exercise

Physical activity falls into four basic categories and the best exercise regimen includes exercise from each group. The four basic exercise categories are endurance, strength, balance, and flexibility.

Endurance exercises, which include jogging, dancing, swimming, brisk walking, and biking, increase your breathing and get your heart pumping. These exercises keep your heart, lungs, and circulatory system healthy and contribute to reduced risk of chronic diseases like diabetes and heart disease.

Strength training, which involves lifting weights or using resistance bands, improves your muscle mass and just makes you a stronger person overall.

Balance exercises, like tai chi, help prevent falls and improve balance, while flexibility exercises, like yoga, stretch your muscles and keep you limber.

Yoga for Your Gut

While all types of exercise are important, yoga may be particularly beneficial for gut health. Since ancient times, yogis have understood that proper digestion is the answer to good health. Yogis also realize that there is a strong mind-body connection, which means that any stress or emotions you're dealing with will show up in your gut.

Some examples of conditions that yogis believe are caused by stress include:

- Diarrhea
- Constipation
- Nausea
- Stomach ulcers
- Celiac disease

- Indigestion
- Esophageal spasms
- Irritable bowel syndrome

Yoga works on digestion and gut health in two ways: by calming the mind to restore normal digestion and by stretching the soft tissues to allow waste material to move through the digestive system properly. When you experience high levels of chronic stress, it negatively affects all areas of digestion, from the excretion of digestive fluids to the contraction of intestinal muscles.

On the flip side, relaxation helps promote healthy digestion. The deep breathing and "be here now" philosophy of yoga is meant to help quiet the mind to reduce the effects of stress on the digestive system.

ESSENTIAL

There are some yoga poses that are thought to be particularly helpful for promoting healthy digestion. These poses include Cat Stretch, Lazy Dog, Extended Child Pose, Downward-Facing Dog, Cow Pose, and Flowing Standard Forward Fold.

The bending and posing in yoga also work like a gentle massage on the soft tissues. When you hold a yoga pose, it compresses the organs of the digestive system. This encourages the contraction of muscles in the digestive system and the movement of previously stagnant fluids and waste materials. Once the waste materials start moving through the digestive tract, you can eliminate them more easily.

Starting a Routine and Preventing Boredom

If you haven't exercised in years, you should check with your physician before you begin any routine. According to most doctors, as long as you do not have a heart condition, you can start working out, but it is important that you check in first. In addition, you may find your healthcare provider has some good ideas, suggestions, and resources to help you start a routine.

Start Slowly

Starting an exercise routine is never easy, so start slowly and be gentle as you work into a routine. (This is especially true if you can't remember the last time you broke a sweat on purpose.) Choose one activity to perform regularly to increase the amount of exercise you get. Start doing it, then add something else, as variety will keep you challenged, and help you keep with it. Encourage your family, friends, or significant other to join you.

Set Goals

It feels good to set new goals and reach them. Whether you want to exercise four times a week for 30 minutes a day or walk 1 mile in 15 minutes, setting goals can keep you motivated. The only caveat: set goals that are reasonable and attainable. Don't set yourself up to fail. If your goals are unattainable, you can lose motivation when you don't meet them. It's unrealistic to think that you're going to go from a coach potato to running a 5K in one month. Set small goals and be proud of yourself when you reach each one.

Reward Yourself

Even if it's a pat on the back, tell yourself what a fantastic job you're doing. Once you master a yoga pose that you thought would be impossible, reward yourself with new workout gear or even a pedicure. Be your own best cheerleader! Beginning to exercise is no small feat and every step you take in the right direction is a step toward balancing your gut and feeling better.

Ban Boredom

One of the most common reasons people quit exercising is boredom. It is easy to fall into a rut when you're doing the same routine day after day. Be intentional about varying your routine from time to time. Walk outside one day and hit the pool at your gym the next. Take a yoga class outside or sign up for salsa dancing. The key to sticking with an exercise routine is to keep things interesting. Make exercise something you want to do, not something you have to do. Encourage a friend to exercise with you. You can take a class together or go walking on a hiking trail.

Take Care

When you have gut health issues, you need to factor some considerations into your exercise plan. Avoid eating for 2 hours prior to exercise—especially anything fatty, gas-producing, or anything you've experienced problems with in the past. If you do eat before you exercise, keep track of your portions: A large meal will require 2–3 hours of digestion before exercise, while a smaller snack may require only 30–60 minutes. Avoid caffeine or hot drinks before exercising; they have the potential to increase abdominal cramping. Try to time your workouts so you exercise at the times when your intestines are quieter, like in the morning before breakfast or between lunch and dinner.

CHAPTER 8

Children and Gut Health

If your child's digestive system isn't working well, his overall health will suffer. Poor eating habits don't just cause temporary digestive distress in little ones. The long-term health risks for a variety of conditions increase, as well. Dr. Elizabeth Lipski explains in *Digestive Wellness for Children*, "Digestive problems are directly linked to a slew of seemingly unrelated juvenile illnesses including arthritis, attention deficit disorders, autism, migraines, asthma, depression, diabetes, and more." Parents and caregivers can recognize digestive factors in children's health and behavioral concerns, find solutions, and encourage healthier habits for the entire family. Creating good digestive health begins early.

Children and Good Gut Health

Good gut health is important for everyone, but it's especially critical for children. Children are constantly growing. As they grow, their immune systems develop, new cells form, and their brains expand. Because children get all the nutrients needed to grow and develop from their gut, having a healthy gut is vital to their success. An unhealthy gut can cause a host of problems.

Gut Health and Autism

The term *autism* is a general name for a group of complex brain disorders. The thing that autism disorders have in common is they involve difficulties in social interaction and communication, both verbal and nonverbal. Children with autism also often engage in repetitive behaviors like repeating words and phrases or asking the same question over and over again. There are varying degrees of autism that fall onto what is called the autism spectrum.

FACT

The Centers for Disease Control and Prevention estimates that 1 in every 68 children in the United States has autism. This is a tenfold increase in autism prevalence in the last 40 years. Boys are four times more likely to have autism than girls.

Another similarity among children with autism is that many of them have a history of requiring long-term or recurrent antibiotic therapy and they usually suffer from gastrointestinal problems like abdominal pain, constipation, diarrhea, and bloating. This leads many researchers to hypothesize that gut health, specifically an imbalance in the good and bad bacteria, may be at least partially to blame.

Immunity and Gut Health

As with adults, a child's gastrointestinal system is the first line of defense for the immune system. When the health of the gut is compromised because of antibiotics, sugary foods, or medications, your child becomes more susceptible to illness and infection.

Mood

Serotonin is a chemical created by your body that works as a neurotransmitter, sending messages between the body and the brain. Serotonin is produced by both the brain and the intestines, but the large majority—80–90 percent—is found in the gut. This neurotransmitter has an effect on mood, social behavior, sleep patterns, and memory, among other things. If the balance of bacteria in your child's gut gets thrown off, it can lead to depressed moods, behavioral problems, and disruptions in sleeping patterns.

Getting Started on the Right Path

The best thing a woman can do to contribute to her child's gut health is to breastfeed her infant. This helps ensure a healthy development of the intestinal tract and immune system by introducing a diverse supply of beneficial bacteria. Breastmilk also contains a variety of antibodies that the immune system uses to fight off infections and disease from bacteria, viruses, and toxins. Eventually humans produce their own antibodies but in the early stages of life, a mother's breastmilk is the only source of antibodies for a baby.

ESSENTIAL

If there are obstacles that prevent a mother from breastfeeding, she can help ensure a healthy balance of bacteria in her baby's gut by supplementing with probiotics. The best supplement is one made for infants that contains a mix of beneficial bacteria.

If your child is older and breastfeeding is no longer relevant, you can still promote gut health and healthy digestion through the practice of healthy habits.

Planning for Optimal Gut Health

Your child's good digestive health begins at home. From what you buy, prepare, and serve to your family's activity level, you can play a significant role in how healthy your child is. Almost every family can make improvements in their diet or lifestyle to encourage better eating habits and health.

Dr. Sarah Ballantyne, the face behind "The Paleo Mom," says that the two most important things you can do to foster healthy eating habits in your child are to eat healthily yourself and to offer him healthy food options; however, even if you know what's right for your child, getting him to eat it is another story.

ESSENTIAL

Don't give up if your child refuses a new fruit or veggie. According to the American Academy of Pediatrics, many children will not accept a new food until it has been offered at least ten times. Continue to offer new foods until your child considers them familiar.

The best thing to do is to start healthy habits early, but even if your child is a little older, you can still instill healthy habits. The key is to approach the situation with patience.

Avoid Gut Irritants

The first thing to do to ensure optimal gut health for your child is remove or limit anything in the diet that causes irritation to the gut. The foods most likely to cause gut irritation are grains, dairy, refined sugars, and processed foods. Processed food often contains a wide variety of ingredients including artificial flavors, artificial sweeteners, coloring agents, MSG, and many more. Your child's body doesn't recognize these chemicals and instead of processing them like food, it processes them like a potentially dangerous item. If a child's body is repeatedly exposed to these artificial ingredients, it can cause damage to the gut.

It's also important to remove any foods that your child may be sensitive or intolerant to. Sensitivities to nuts, eggs, seeds, and nightshade vegetables, which include tomatoes, peppers, and eggplants, are some of the most common among children. If you're unsure about whether your child is sensitive to a particular food, you can ask your naturopath or functional medicine doctor to order food sensitivity tests. If the test shows any food sensitivities, eliminate that item from the diet as well. You can also identify the presence of any food sensitivities by putting your child on an elimination diet; however, putting your child on a strict elimination diet can be difficult, especially if he eats lunch at school or goes to friends' houses regularly.

Buy Organic Produce Whenever Possible

In terms of relative body weight, children consume more pesticides than adults. The problem is that their bodies aren't prepared to cope with it. Because children's detoxification systems aren't fully developed, they are much more likely to accumulate chemicals over a longer period of time and in greater amounts.

Combined with the fact that children are often picky eaters and may eat only a few specific fruits or vegetables, they are more than likely ingesting one particular pesticide or group of pesticides in larger amounts. Unfortunately, this can lead to toxic levels rather easily in a small body as chemicals accumulate in muscle or fat tissue.

If you can't afford to buy all of your produce organic or you don't have access to organics, use the Environmental Working Group's Dirty Dozen Plus list to determine which foods are most important to buy organic. The Dirty Dozen Plus list includes the fourteen foods that contain the highest amount of pesticides, even after washing.

Foods on the Dirty Dozen Plus list include (listed from highest to lowest):

- Apples
- Strawberries
- Grapes
- Celery
- Peaches
- Spinach
- Sweet bell peppers
- Nectarines (imported)
- Cucumbers
- Cherry tomatoes
- Snap peas (imported)
- Potatoes
- Hot peppers
- Blueberries (domestic)

Many organic foods are also more nutrient dense than their conventional counterparts. Supplying your child with nutrient-dense food will help support his rapid growth and development.

In addition to the Dirty Dozen Plus list, the Environmental Working Group also created the Clean Fifteen list, which includes the fifteen fruits and vegetables that contain the lowest amount of pesticides. If you have to budget your spending or have limited produce access, these are the best conventional choices.

Produce on the Clean Fifteen list includes:

- Avocados
- Sweet corn
- Pineapples
- Cabbage
- Sweet peas (frozen)
- Onions
- Asparagus
- Mangoes
- Papayas
- Kiwi
- Eggplant
- Grapefruit
- Cantaloupe
- Cauliflower
- Sweet potatoes

Aim for a Healthy Weight

For children, being overweight is a significant health concern. More than one-third of children are considered overweight or obese. Overweight children are more likely to be overweight teens, who are more likely to be overweight adults. The health risks associated with child obesity are serious. Children who weigh too much are more likely to develop heart disease, type 2 diabetes, some types of cancer, joint problems, and more. There's also a psychological impact of obesity for kids who don't feel good about their size. Obesity tends to decrease self-esteem and disrupt social growth.

ESSENTIAL

Studies have shown that disruptions in gut flora may increase the rate at which fatty acids and carbohydrates are absorbed. An unhealthy gut balance may also increase the amount of calories your child stores as fat.

Help your child reach or stay at a healthy weight by encouraging healthy eating habits and regular movement. Get your child involved in sports or outdoor play and limit time in front of the television or computer. Stress the consumption of vegetables and reduce exposure to refined sugars and unhealthy fatty foods.

QUESTION

What's a fast snack I can keep in the refrigerator for the kids?
Make turkey roll-ups without the bread. Top a piece of freshly roasted turkey meat with a slice of avocado, a pickle spear, and a dollop of mustard. Roll up the piece of turkey and secure with a toothpick. Keep a few ready in the fridge for hunger emergencies.

Here are some other tips for helping your children eat healthy:

- Model good eating yourself.
- Add new healthy recipes to your list of tried-and-true ones.
- Plan healthy eating for the whole family.
- Make mealtimes a pleasure and never give food as a reward or withhold food as a punishment.
- Offer a wide range of fresh foods to make sure kids get all the nutrients they need.
- Invite children to help with choosing and cooking food. You'll be giving them a healthy attitude toward food that will last a lifetime.
- Limit fast food.

Avoid Refined Sugar

Refined sugar has no nutritional benefit. Not only that, but it actually promotes poor health in your child as well. Refined sugar contributes to widespread inflammation, which damages the gut lining, setting your child up for chronic health problems, like heart disease and problems with cholesterol. Refined sugar also contributes to irritability and the formation of cavities.

A report from the Centers for Disease Control and Prevention found that the average child gets about 16 percent of his calories from refined sugar. Most of the added sugar comes from processed, nutrient-poor foods, and soft drinks. A child can take in 10 teaspoons' worth of sugar just from drinking one can of soda. The report went on to add that most calories from added sugar were consumed inside the home, not at school or a friend's house.

It's best to remove added sugar from your child's diet completely, although that might be unrealistic since you can't control everything that goes into your child's mouth outside of the home. Reduce your child's intake of added sugar by keeping soft drinks and sugar-laden cereals and snacks out of the house. Provide fresh fruit as a snack or dessert after dinner instead of ice cream or cookies.

Watch Out for School Lunches

While your child's school may offer healthier lunches, that doesn't mean your child is going to choose them. Often, the same schools that tout healthy alternatives fail to mention that hot dogs, fries, and ice cream are still on the daily menu and easily accessible. Unless your child's school is committed to providing organic, whole foods, start sending your child off with a packed lunch.

Many children consume at least half of their meals at school. Unfortunately, menus served in school lunch programs are often full of processed, frozen foods and are too low in fiber- and nutrient-rich fruit and vegetables. Encourage your child to make healthier choices by teaching the importance of proper nutrition.

Get your child involved in the process by allowing him to choose a few items while grocery shopping and encouraging him to help you pack the lunch. Children are more likely to actually eat what's in a healthy lunch bag if they are at least partly involved in choosing the menu and preparing the meal. You don't have to give your child free reign, but offer a choice between carrot sticks or cut-up cucumbers and cherries or grapes. Skip prepackaged lunches. Very few of them are healthy and most are more expensive than what you can prepare on your own.

Respect Your Child's Choices

For children, food is a form of sustenance. As a general rule, they'll eat when they're hungry and pass when they're not. Respect your child's ability to determine whether or not she wants to eat. Don't force food or create arguments at the table. This can cause an unhealthy relationship with food and lead your child to associate mealtime with anxiety, stress, and frustration. On the other hand, don't use food as a reward. A child shouldn't learn to eat broccoli because if she does she'll get dessert. She should learn to eat it because it's good for her and she'll like it.

Have Fun

Play time is not only important for a child's developing brain, it also helps regulate hormones, including the stress hormones that play a role in gut health. Make time to play with your child. Set up play dates with other children. Vary types of play. One day you might decide to play soccer, while another day you decide to play a board game or put together a puzzle.

Get Outside

In addition to the fresh air and open play environment the outdoors provides, it also allows your children to be exposed to sunlight, which aids in the production of vitamin D. Vitamin D is essential for reducing inflammation and promoting healing, two characteristics that are crucial to gut health. There are very few sources of vitamin D in the diet, so sun exposure is particularly important, especially if you live in a climate that doesn't see the sun all year long. Aim to get outside before noon or after 2 P.M., when the sun is at its peak, to avoid sunburn.

When Problems Arise

Digestive conditions are often more common during childhood than adult-hood. Plus, many digestive diseases start in childhood and progress into adulthood. If the digestive problems are not diagnosed and treated in child-hood, there can be long-term health consequences.

Children and Diarrhea

At some point, all children get diarrhea. Loose, watery, soft, or more frequent bowel movements are most commonly associated with a stom-ach virus, especially if it is also accompanied with vomiting and low-grade fever. While uncomfortable, occasional bouts are not dangerous. It usually resolves in a day or two and may be related to a change in diet or anxiety.

Diarrhea can be dangerous in newborns and infants. In small children, severe diarrhea lasting just a day or two can lead to dehydration. Rotavirus is a common virus that can make small children ill very quickly. Because a child can die from dehydration within a few days, the main treatment for diarrhea in children is rehydration.

Most cases of diarrhea in children are caused by viruses and will clear up on their own, according to Dr. Joseph Croffie, director of the Gas-trointestinal Motility Laboratory at Riley Hospital for Children in Indi-anapolis. Parents can ensure that their children are getting enough fluids by encouraging them to sip water frequently.

Call your child's healthcare provider if any of the following symptoms appear:

- Stools containing blood or pus, or black stools
- Temperature above 101.4°F
- No improvement after 24 hours
- Signs of dehydration (dry mouth and tongue; no tears when crying; sunken abdomen, eyes, or cheeks; listlessness or irritability; or skin that does not flatten when pinched and released)

If your child experiences chronic diarrhea that does not seem to go away, you may be dealing with a food sensitivity or intolerance. In this case, it may be beneficial to work with a functional medicine doctor who can order proper testing to get to the underlying cause.

Constipation Tips

Constipation is fairly common among children. Once children are over a year old, many have bowel movements once a day. Almost all children have occasional bouts of constipation. Postponing a toilet trip until after an activity or favorite show may lead to constipation problems later on. Teach your child to go when she feels the urge and not to hold it.

Home Treatment for Constipation

Treating constipation in children is similar to treating constipation in adults. Increased fluids, exercise, and a high-fiber diet will all help prevent and treat constipation. Improving those areas will usually be beneficial enough on their own. Heavy intake of dairy products (even just 2–3 cups of milk a day) may also create constipation. If your child is experiencing chronic constipation, cut back on dairy and see how the bowels respond.

Preventing Food Allergies

Discuss the timing of food introduction with your child's healthcare provider. Frequently, early exposure may lead to an increased likelihood of problems. Parents are often excited about progressing to solid food, but if this is done too soon it may end up creating a food sensitivity or intolerance.

CHAPTER 9

Knowing When to Seek Help

If you're experiencing chronic symptoms, like regular head-aches, fatigue, constipation, and/or heartburn, you're not alone. In fact, you're in the company of millions of others. Just because chronic symptoms are common, however, doesn't mean you should accept living with them. You don't have to deal with ailments that interfere with your day-to-day life or put up with symptoms that disrupt your quality of life. Even, and especially, if you've been to a traditional medical doctor who has given you a clean bill of health or told you your symptoms are all in your head, it's time to find someone who can help you get rid of your symptoms and live the quality of life you deserve.

Finding a Doctor Who Can Help

In the traditional healthcare model, a doctor looks at the symptoms you're experiencing and then prescribes medication to help get rid of the symptoms. The problem with this technique is that while the medication may suppress symptoms, it doesn't always address the underlying cause of the symptoms. Eventually, the symptoms return with a vengeance or new symptoms will pop up in their place.

ALERT

Many medications are not only ineffective at getting rid of the underlying cause of symptoms, but they also come with a host of potential side effects. While many medications come with a list of known side effects, many side effects don't become known until after the drug has officially hit the market.

Not only that, but this healthcare model also generally requires that you're on medication for the rest of your life—or at least for a very long time. The key to eliminating symptoms for good is to figure out the deeper cause, the physiological imbalance that's causing the symptoms in the first place. This is where functional medicine comes in.

Functional Medicine

Many people who turn to functional medicine have already undergone several diagnostic tests and blood tests under the traditional healthcare model without finding any answers as to what might be ailing them. Oftentimes, these test results will come back normal. If you've been experiencing chronic symptoms and have yet to find any answers or relief, you may want to consider working with a functional medicine practitioner.

Functional medicine is a patient-centered approach to healthcare that focuses on the individual as a person instead of isolating symptoms or diagnosing a specific disease. The belief behind functional medicine is that a symptomatic disease, like diabetes, chronic fatigue syndrome, fibromyalgia, or cancer, is only the tip of the iceberg. Symptoms are meant to alert your body that there's some type of altered physiology below the surface. This altered physiology may be in the form of hormonal imbalances, immune imbalances, exposure to toxic chemicals, or digestive and gut imbalance. The key to optimal health is restoring homeostasis—internal stability—by identifying and fixing any imbalances.

ESSENTIAL

You can find a functional medicine practitioner near you by going to the Institute for Functional Medicine's website at *www.functional medicine.org* and clicking on the "Find a Practitioner" link. Here you can search by name, practice, specialty, degree, or location. The practitioners listed in the IFM database have successfully passed the IFM's certification program.

Basic Principles

The guiding principle behind functional medicine is that all treatment should be patient-centered. This means that your functional medicine practitioner will focus on you as a unique individual. All decisions regarding treatment will take your needs, values, and preferences into consideration. The theory behind this principle is that making you an active participant in your health will give you more of a sense of control and allow you to sustain the lifestyle changes that are necessary for you to reach optimal health.

QUESTION

What if I don't agree with something the doctor wants me to do?
The beauty of functional medicine is that your doctor makes you an active partner in your health and your treatment plan. If you're unsure of something your doctor suggests or you want to go a different route, speak up. Your doctor will take your feelings into consideration. If he doesn't, find a new one.

Functional medicine is also based largely on the fact that every individual is unique on a biochemical level. This means that even if you're experiencing the same symptoms as someone else, the reason or under-lying imbalance may be completely different, and therefore, the treatment approach must be completely different as well. A functional medicine practitioner realizes that true health is not merely the absence of disease. In order to reach true vitality, you must be emotionally, physically, and spiritually fulfilled. An imbalance in one area can cause a great deal of dysfunction in another area.

An Integrative Approach

Integrative medicine is about treating the whole person. It recognizes that the person is not just a physical being and, therefore, instead of only treating the body, it focuses on mind and spirit as well. Integrative medicine combines some of the theories of mainstream medicine with complementary and alternative therapies.

In order to get the full effect from integrative medicine, it's often necessary to involve a whole team of skilled practitioners. This may mean that in order to reach optimal gut health, you need a functional medicine doctor, a nutritionist, a massage therapist, and an acupuncturist on board. You may need to practice meditation with a skilled Buddhist or do regular yoga with a trained yoga instructor.

FACT

The term *complementary* refers to the practice of using nonmainstream approaches to a condition in addition to conventional medicine. The term *alternative* describes using nonmainstream approaches instead of conventional medicine. An integrative approach considers all available options and uses the best combination to treat the person.

When you start working with a functional medicine practitioner, she will usually have recommendations for other healthcare practitioners for you to go see. Once your treatment plan has been outlined, she will be able to point you in the right direction. Some functional medicine practitioners work in centers with other healthcare professionals so that you have easy access to other professionals who can help you on your journey to optimal health.

What's Involved in Treatment

Once your functional medicine doctor identifies the imbalances that are causing your symptoms, you and he will work together to develop a treatment plan. Treatment is comprehensive and focuses on correcting the imbalance by addressing every area—body, mind, and spirit.

ALERT

As your health progresses and your symptoms improve, your treatment plan might change. It is important to go to regular follow-up appointments with your functional medicine doctor to keep track of your progress and assess whether any changes need to be made.

Treatment may consist of therapeutic diets, nutritional supplements, botanical medicines, or detoxification programs. In some cases, medication might be necessary to control symptoms while your doctor works with you to correct the imbalances. Your treatment program may also include counseling, regular exercise, and incorporating stress-management techniques like meditation, yoga, and deep breathing.

Preparing for Your Appointment

Because your first appointment with a functional medicine doctor is so comprehensive, you'll often be asked to do some preparation in advance. After you make your appointment, the doctor's office may send you new-patient forms to fill out. These forms cover all areas, from your medical history to your social life, so they are often several pages long. Fill out the forms completely and accurately to save time once you get to your appointment.

You may also want to gather all your previous medical test results and make a list of current medications, supplements, or vitamins that you're taking. It's often helpful to write down a list of questions you may have or concerns that you want addressed in advance so that you don't forget anything during your appointment. Arrive to your appointment at least 15 minutes early so the receptionist can look over your intake forms and give you any new forms that you may need to fill out.

What to Expect at Your Appointment

Your appointment with a functional medicine doctor will differ greatly from the appointments you're used to having with a traditional medical doctor. Traditional doctors are often only allotted a certain amount of time to see each patient. This is about 8 minutes, on average. That's it. You may feel rushed and leave feeling like your questions weren't adequately answered. When you see a functional medicine doctor, you will have a comprehensive appointment that will include a medical history, physical examination, and possible laboratory testing. An initial appointment with a functional medicine doctor may last an hour.

Your functional medicine doctor will ask you for a detailed description of your medical history. She will ask if you've been diagnosed with any illnesses, if there's a history of specific illnesses in your family, and what symptoms, if any, you're currently experiencing. In addition to asking for a physical medical history, she will also ask questions about your spiritual health, mental well-being, and social life. She'll want to know how much you exercise, where your water comes from, what type of diet you follow, and whether you're exposed to any environmental pollutants or toxins.

You may have to answer some of the following questions:

- Are you happy with your weight?
- Would you describe yourself as happy?
- Do you like your job?
- How would you describe your stress level?
- Do you handle stress well?
- Do you have trouble falling asleep?
- Do you feel like your life has meaning?
- Do you have a close social circle?
- Do you feel safe at home?
- Do you ever feel the need to hide your eating?
- How often do you laugh?

These questions aren't meant to pry into your personal life, but rather to get the whole story about you as a person. The answers to these questions give your functional medicine doctor clues about your physical, emotional, and spiritual health and help the doctor recommend the best path when it comes to restoring vitality and getting you on the road to optimal health. It's important to answer each question honestly and thoroughly. There is no need to hold back or feel embarrassed about any of your answers. The doctor is not there to judge; she is there to help.

Functional Medicine and Gut Health

Now that you know what functional medicine is, you may be wondering why it's important to gut health. Having a healthy gut is the cornerstone of health. Your gut is connected to your entire body. Dr. Mark Hyman, one of the leading functional medicine practitioners, says that when someone comes to him with a chronic health problem, such as allergies, autoimmune diseases, cancer, or chronic fatigue syndrome, the first thing he does is work to fix the gut. A traditional doctor may not realize that conditions like eczema or arthritis, which seem totally unrelated to the gut, actually stem from gut dysfunction.

It's important to work with someone who understands how important gut health is to the overall health of your body and what the necessary steps are to fix it.

Functional Medicine Testing

The Western model of medicine focuses on disease, while functional medicine focuses on wellness. When a medical doctor orders lab tests, he is looking for the telltale signs of an existing disease. For example, high glucose levels may indicate diabetes, while low thyroid hormone levels may point to hypothyroidism. If there are no definite disease markers, a medical doctor will assume that there are no health problems; however, if you're experiencing chronic symptoms, you know there is something going on whether or not a traditional test shows it. This is where functional medicine lab testing comes in.

Functional medicine doctors do not treat diseases; they work to understand what is causing symptoms and then correct the underlying imbalance. A functional medicine doctor looks for imbalances that may cause symptoms, but have not gotten to the point where an actual "disease" is present.

In order to identify or rule out any imbalances, your functional medicine doctor may order a series of lab tests.

QUESTION

Will my insurance cover the lab testing ordered by a functional medicine practitioner?
The amount of coverage you have for functional lab testing depends on your insurance company. Many tests are not covered. Before you go for any testing, contact your insurance company and ask about coverage so you're not surprised if you get a bill from the lab.

Some of these lab tests, like blood testing, may resemble traditional lab testing, while others, like stool testing and hair analysis, are more unique to the functional medicine practice. Each test gives your doctor clues about your current state of health and the steps he must take to restore normal functioning.

Functional Blood Chemistry Analysis

When your medical doctor orders a traditional blood test, he is looking for the absence of disease. If everything appears normal in that regard, you're given a clean bill of health. A functional blood chemistry analysis goes deeper. Your functional medicine doctor looks at patterns that may indicate metabolic imbalances that may be causing symptoms or can eventually lead to disease. A functional blood chemistry analysis will give your functional medicine doctor clues about all areas of your health including:

- Gut health
- Adrenals and kidney health
- Thyroid health
- Immune health
- Nutrient deficiencies
- Toxicity
- Inflammation

Generally, a blood chemistry analysis is one of the first tests your functional medicine doctor will order. Once the results from the blood analysis come in, your doctor will have more clues as to which direction he should go. This often means more comprehensive lab testing.

Stool Analysis

Stool testing is used to identify imbalances of bacteria, yeast, or parasites in the gut. When you have an overgrowth of bacteria or too much yeast in the digestive tract, it can lead to gastrointestinal symptoms like gas, bloating, constipation, diarrhea, and heartburn. Imbalances in the gut are also often the cause of chronic inflammation, malnutrition, chronic fatigue, mental disorders, and autoimmune diseases. Your functional medicine doctor can use a stool analysis to determine if you have problems with yeast, an overgrowth of bacteria, or unwanted parasites.

ESSENTIAL

Your doctor will usually request a minimum of three stool samples on three separate days to maximize detection of possible parasitic infections. You'll generally collect these samples at home and either bring them in to your doctor to send to the lab or send them to the lab directly in sanitary packaging that's provided to you.

In addition to identifying any unwanted bugs, a stool analysis can also tell your doctor if you have an inflammation in your intestinal tract, if you're having problems absorbing fats, and if you're sensitive to any medications that you're taking.

Saliva Analysis

Many functional medicine doctors prefer saliva testing over blood testing because a saliva test measures active, bio-available hormones, whereas a blood test measures only inactive hormones. With an accuracy rating of 92–96 percent, saliva tests are also considered more accurate than blood tests; and as an added bonus, they're noninvasive. Saliva can be collected anytime and anywhere. A saliva test measures the levels of various hormones, including cortisol, estrogen, progesterone, testosterone, and DHEA. Testing your hormonal levels gives your functional medicine doctor clues about your adrenal health and thyroid health, among other things.

Food Sensitivity Testing

Food allergies trigger the immune system to release histamine, which is responsible for the characteristic symptoms of an allergic response. The symptoms of a food allergy come on quickly and can be life threatening in those with severe allergies. A true allergic reaction is mediated by Immunoglobulin E or IgE. In order to diagnosis a food allergy, doctors may use skin testing or a blood test called RAST to identify the presence of IgE. True food allergies affect approximately 3–4 percent of the population.

Traditional food allergy testing cannot diagnose food sensitivities, which are much more common than true food allergies, because food sensitivities are mediated by Immunoglobulin G or IgG. Instead of producing an immediate response, IgG reactions take several hours to several days to develop. Because it can take so long for a food sensitivity to produce a symptom, it often goes undiagnosed. An undiagnosed food sensitivity can do a great deal of damage to the gut and lead to many chronic health problems.

In order to test for a food sensitivity, your functional medicine doctor may request an IgG food sensitivity profile. This test measures your reaction to 30–200 different foods, depending on the specific test. IgG food sensitivity profiles require you to give blood.

Hair Mineral Analysis

A hair mineral analysis measures the levels of 20 minerals and toxic metals in the hair, but it does so much more than that. An analysis of the hair can give your functional medicine doctor important clues about your energy levels, metabolic rate, stress levels, immune function, and tolerance to sugars and carbohydrates. Although the hair is dead tissue, it stores information about the mineral activity that took place over a period of 3–4 months. Analyzing the hair allows your doctor to determine whether your gut is absorbing the minerals you need from the food you eat and can also let your doctor know if there's a metal toxicity present that may be interfering with your gut health.

Toxic metals are easier to detect in the hair than in the blood because the body moves them quickly from the blood to soft tissues, like the hair, where they can't do as much damage to the body as a whole. Hair testing also allows a more long-term reading, while blood and urine tests are more a measure of what is going on in the body at that specific moment in time.

Neurotransmitter Profile

The neurotransmitter profile measures the level of the six main neurotransmitters: serotonin, dopamine, GABA, glutamate, adrenaline, and noradrenaline. As you now know, most of the serotonin—the neurotransmitter responsible for your mood—is produced in your gut. Testing your neurotransmitters can give your functional medicine doctor clues about what's going on in your gut and how your gut health may be influencing your mood, sleep, hormones, appetite, and cognitive function.

The Institute for Functional Medicine notes that many functional imbalances can be completely restored, while others can be greatly improved. It's ideal to start working with a functional medicine doctor before a chronic disease state begins. Prevention is easier than reversal.

CHAPTER 10

Breakfast and Brunch

Easy Pancakes

This pancake recipe is quick and easy and can be multiplied to make enough for an entire family. Once cooked, sprinkle the pancake with cinnamon for an old-fashioned pancake taste.

INGREDIENTS | SERVES 1

1 large ripe banana
1 large egg
1 tablespoon nut butter of choice
2 teaspoons coconut oil

Bananas As Thickeners

Bananas can be a good replacement for flour when you're trying to avoid wheat and gluten. Bananas act as a thickening agent in recipes that would normally be too fluid.

1. In a small bowl, mash banana with a fork.

2. Beat egg and add to banana.

3. Add nut butter and mix well.

4. Heat oil in a small frying pan or griddle over medium heat. Pour all pancake batter onto preheated pan.

5. Cook until lightly brown on each side, about 2 minutes per side.

PER SERVING | Calories: 368 | Fat: 23 g | Protein: 11 g | Sodium: 104 mg | Fiber: 7 g | Carbohydrates: 35 g | Sugar: 18 g

Fluffy Coconut Pancakes

If you have gone gluten-free, one of the things you may miss is a good pancake breakfast. These pancakes are gluten-free and go great with fresh fruit.

INGREDIENTS | SERVES 4 (2 PANCAKES PER SERVING)

3 large eggs

¾ cup coconut milk

½ teaspoon all-natural sea salt

3 tablespoons melted coconut oil, divided

½ cup coconut flour, sifted

1 teaspoon baking powder

1. Mix eggs, coconut milk, salt, and 2 tablespoons melted coconut oil in a large bowl.

2. Thoroughly combine coconut flour and baking powder in a small bowl. Mix into batter. The mixture will be thin at first, but the coconut flour will absorb the liquid and the batter will thicken as stirred. The batter will be thick and will flatten out as the pancakes cook.

3. In a heavy-bottomed skillet, heat remaining coconut oil on medium heat.

4. Scoop batter onto skillet, using ¼ cup measuring cup for each pancake. Cook for about 1 minute, then turn. Cook for another minute, or until cooked through and golden brown.

5. For waffles, scoop batter into a well-oiled waffle iron and follow cooking directions.

PER SERVING | Calories: 290 | Fat: 25 g | Protein: 8 g | Sodium: 480 mg | Fiber: 0 g | Carbohydrates: 6 g | Sugar: 1 g

Strawberry-Banana Pancakes

These pancakes are a great alternative to eggs, which tend to be the go-to grain-free breakfast choice.

INGREDIENTS | SERVES 1

2 teaspoons coconut oil
3 large egg whites, lightly beaten
1 large banana, sliced
4 strawberries, sliced
1 tablespoon melted almond butter
⅛ teaspoon ground cinnamon

1. Preheat a small frying pan, add coconut oil, and swirl to coat pan.

2. Combine egg whites, banana, strawberries, and almond butter in a medium bowl and mix well.

3. Pour into pan, cover with lid, and cook for about 2–3 minutes, until bottom is golden brown.

4. Flip pancake to brown the other side, 2–3 minutes.

5. Serve warm with cinnamon sprinkled on top.

PER SERVING | Calories: 316 | Fat: 10 g | Protein: 19 g | Sodium: 230 mg | Fiber: 7 g | Carbohydrates: 40 g | Sugar: 21 g

Homemade Almond Milk

Because homemade almond milk doesn't contain any artificial preservatives, it has a shorter shelf life than the almond milk you purchase in the store. Only make what you plan to drink in 2–3 days.

INGREDIENTS | MAKES 2 CUPS (1-CUP SERVINGS)

1 cup unsalted almonds
2 cups filtered water

1. Place almonds in a small bowl and cover with water. Let soak, uncovered, for 8–12 hours or overnight.

2. After 8–12 hours, drain soaking water into a blender and rinse almonds.

3. Add rinsed almonds to the blender with soaking water and blend for 2 minutes.

4. Place nut bag or cheesecloth over a container and pour blended almond mixture into the nut bag or cheesecloth.

5. Twist nut bag or cheesecloth and squeeze the contents, allowing all of the liquid to seep into the container. Store covered in refrigerator for up to 3 days.

6. For vanilla almond milk, place 2 pitted dates and 1 teaspoon of real vanilla extract in the blender with almonds and soaking water.

PER SERVING | Calories: 46 | Fat: 4 g | Protein: 1 g | Sodium: 4 mg | Fiber: 1 g | Carbohydrates: 1 g | Sugar: 0 g

Fruity Egg Frittata

This delicious blend of fruit atop a light and fluffy egg frittata makes a surprisingly sweet breakfast treat. Light, but packed full of protein, this breakfast will rev up your day without weighing you down.

INGREDIENTS | SERVES 5

Coconut oil
1 cup sliced strawberries
1 cup blueberries
1 cup raspberries
10 large eggs
1 teaspoon vanilla extract

Essential Vanilla Extract

When a recipe calls for vanilla, use *real* vanilla extract. Although real vanilla extract is more expensive than imitation, the flavor is far superior. Store vanilla extract in a cool, dark place to preserve the flavor.

1. Preheat oven to 350°F. Coat a 10" oven-safe frying pan with coconut oil.

2. Over medium heat, sauté all fruit together until lightly heated and softened.

3. While fruit is heating, briskly whisk together egg whites and vanilla until well blended. Add to prepared frying pan, covering fruit completely.

4. Continue cooking until the center solidifies slightly and bubbles begin to appear, 2–3 minutes.

5. Remove from heat and place in preheated oven.

6. Cook for 10–15 minutes, or until frittata is firm in the center.

PER SERVING | Calories: 220 | Fat: 12 g | Protein: 15 g | Sodium: 152 mg | Fiber: 3 g | Carbohydrates: 11 g | Sugar: 7 g

Garlicky Veggie-Packed Omelet

Delicious vegetables and garlic combine with fluffy eggs and egg whites to make a simple, satisfying, and savory meal that will start off any day right! Protein-packed and rich in complex carbohydrates from the vegetables, this is a tasty way to get some valuable nutrition.

INGREDIENTS | SERVES 1

2 teaspoons olive oil or coconut oil
¼ cup chopped yellow onion
¼ cup sliced button or cremini mushrooms
2 tablespoons filtered water
½ teaspoon garlic powder
½ cup torn spinach leaves
¼ cup chopped tomato
2 large whole eggs
4 large egg whites

Gracious Garlic

A member of the lily flower family, garlic is a beautiful plant that can give your meal a tantalizing aroma and a unique flavor that can't be found in anything else. Use garlic or garlic powder to dress up dishes, or create a savory flavor.

1. Heat olive oil or coconut oil in a small frying pan over medium heat.

2. Sauté onion for 1 minute. Add mushrooms and water, and sauté until mushrooms are softened, about 3–4 minutes.

3. Sprinkle mixture with garlic powder and add spinach leaves and tomatoes, stirring constantly.

4. Whisk together eggs and egg whites and pour over the sautéed vegetables.

5. Immediately begin pushing the outer edges into the center with a spatula for one turn around the whole pan. Let omelet set for 2 minutes.

6. Gently slide the spatula under omelet and quickly flip.

7. Continue cooking omelet for another 3–5 minutes, or until no longer runny.

PER SERVING | Calories: 357 | Fat: 21 g | Protein: 30 g | Sodium: 375 mg | Fiber: 2 g | Carbohydrates: 10 g | Sugar: 5 g

Very Veggie Frittata

Packed with loads of protein from the egg whites and eggs, and rich in carbohydrates from all of the fresh vegetables, this omelet is both nutritious and delicious. Customize it using your favorite veggies.

INGREDIENTS | SERVES 4

1 tablespoon olive oil or coconut oil

½ cup chopped broccoli

½ cup diced button or cremini mushrooms

½ cup chopped yellow bell pepper

¼ yellow onion, finely chopped

¼ cup filtered water

6 large egg whites

6 large whole eggs

1 teaspoon garlic powder

1 teaspoon all-natural sea salt

2 teaspoons ground black pepper

1. Preheat oven to 350°F. In a large oven-safe skillet, heat olive oil or coconut oil over medium heat.

2. Add broccoli, mushrooms, bell pepper, onion, and water to skillet and cook until tender, but not soft.

3. In a medium bowl, whisk together egg whites, eggs, garlic powder, salt, and pepper and pour over veggie mixture.

4. Cook until the center begins to shake and bubble from the heat, about 3–4 minutes. Remove from heat and place in preheated oven for 10–15 minutes, or until a fork inserted in the center comes out clean.

PER SERVING | Calories: 201 | Fat: 13 g | Protein: 17 g | Sodium: 777 mg | Fiber: 1 g | Carbohydrates: 4 g | Sugar: 2 g

Fresh Fruit Compote

Compotes can be made with a variety of fresh or dried fruit. Delicious fresh fruit that prevent large spikes in blood sugar include stoned fruit such as peaches, plums, apricots, and cherries, or berries such as strawberries, blueberries, blackberries, and raspberries, complemented by citrus fruit such as oranges or tangerines.

INGREDIENTS | SERVES 1

⅛ teaspoon ground cinnamon

⅛ teaspoon vanilla extract

1 cup chopped fresh fruit (such as plums, apricots, or peaches)

Benefits of Fresh Fruit

Fresh fruit not only tastes good, but it also keeps your digestive system moving. A single cup of raspberries contains 8 grams of fiber, almost one-third of your recommendation for the entire day.

Stir cinnamon and vanilla with fruit and enjoy.

PER SERVING | Calories: 77 | Fat: 0 g | Protein: 1 g | Sodium: 0 mg | Fiber: 4 g | Carbohydrates: 19 g | Sugar: 16 g

Old-Fashioned Sweet Potato Hash Browns

These sweet potato hash browns are likely to become a family favorite. They are easy to make and packed with a flavor your entire family will love.

INGREDIENTS | SERVES 6

3 tablespoons coconut oil

3 medium sweet potatoes, peeled and grated

1 teaspoon ground cinnamon

1. Heat coconut oil in a large sauté pan over medium-high heat.

2. Cook sweet potatoes in hot oil for 7 minutes, stirring often.

3. Once browned, sprinkle with cinnamon and serve.

PER SERVING | Calories: 89 | Fat: 2 g | Protein: 1 g | Sodium: 0 mg | Fiber: 2 g | Carbohydrates: 16 g | Sugar: 0 g

Banana-Coconut Bread

This banana-coconut loaf recipe can double as a dessert recipe quite nicely.
Serve with fresh banana and strawberry slices for a delicious treat.

INGREDIENTS | SERVES 8

1¼ cups almond meal

2 teaspoons baking powder

¼ teaspoon baking soda

½ cup fruit purée

¼ teaspoon ground cinnamon

2 large eggs

3 large ripe bananas, mashed

¼ cup flaxseed flour

½ cup chopped walnuts

1 cup unsweetened coconut flakes

Fruit Purées

Fruit purées are a great way to add sweetness to any recipe without using refined sugar. Simply place your favorite fruit into a food processor and quickly pulse to chop finely. You can also use purées in place of syrups and jams.

1. Preheat oven to 350°F. Grease a 9" × 5" loaf pan.

2. Combine almond meal, baking powder, baking soda, fruit purée, cinnamon, eggs, bananas, and flaxseed flour in a large bowl. Mix well.

3. Fold chopped walnuts and coconut flakes into batter (do not overmix). Pour batter into prepared pan.

4. Bake for about 45 minutes or until a wooden toothpick inserted in the center comes out dry.

5. Let bread sit in pan for 5 minutes, then remove from pan and transfer to a wire rack. Let cool completely and serve.

PER SERVING | Calories: 264 | Fat: 12 g | Protein: 6 g | Sodium: 26 mg | Fiber: 6 g | Carbohydrates: 38 g | Sugar: 9 g

Strawberry Dream Smoothie

The perfect combination of clean carbohydrates and protein is packed into this beautiful treat. The simplicity and sweetness of strawberries is sure to make this smoothie a delicious treat for kids and adults alike.

INGREDIENTS | SERVES 2

2 cups strawberries

1 cup full-fat plain kefir

1 teaspoon vanilla extract

1 cup ice, divided

1. Combine strawberries, kefir, and vanilla extract in a blender with ½ cup of the ice, and blend until thoroughly combined.

2. Add remaining ice slowly while blending until desired consistency is reached.

PER SERVING | Calories: 103 | Fat: 3 g | Protein: 5 g | Sodium: 61 mg | Fiber: 2 g | Carbohydrates: 14 g | Sugar: 10 g

Creamy Kefir's Amazing Nutrition

Enjoying a cup of kefir not only loads your mouth with flavor but also packs your body with a ton of nutrition. Brimming with protein that far outweighs that found in milk, you'll reap the benefits of "good" bacteria and enzymes that will optimize your gut health. Kefir is also high in calcium, phosphorus, and vitamin K—three nutrients that are vital to bone health.

Ginger Tea

Ginger has been used for many years in Chinese medicine. It helps alleviate stomach pain, diarrhea, and nausea.

INGREDIENTS | SERVES 4

3 (1") pieces gingerroot
4 cups cold filtered water
Honey or lemon to taste (optional)

1. Peel gingerroot and cut into thin slices.

2. Boil water and add ginger slices.

3. Simmer for 15 minutes.

4. Strain tea and discard ginger slices.

5. Add honey and lemon to taste if desired.

PER SERVING (without honey or lemon) | Calories: 30 | Fat: 0 g | Protein: 0 g | Sodium: 0 mg | Fiber: 0 g | Carbohydrates: 8 g | Sugar: 8 g

Watermelon Orange Juice

This delicious juice reduces cravings for sugary snacks and is great for dumping excess water weight.

INGREDIENTS | SERVES 1 (1½ CUPS)

2 cups watermelon chunks

1 large orange, sectioned

1. Process watermelon and orange through an electronic juicer according to the manufacturer's directions.

2. Serve alone or over ice.

Watermelon for Weight Loss

Watermelon has a diuretic effect. It stimulates your kidneys to dump excess amounts of sodium, which takes water with it. Diuretic foods help you get rid of water weight and help rid the body of toxins.

PER SERVING | Calories: 159 | Fat: 1 g | Protein: 3 g | Sodium: 6 mg | Fiber: 5 g | Carbohydrates: 36 g | Sugar: 20 g

Blueberry Apple Juice

If you prefer, you can add filtered water or serve over ice to dilute this a bit.

1. Process berries through an electronic juicer according to the manufacturer's directions.

2. Add apple, followed by lemon or lime. Process as directed.

3. Stir or shake juice thoroughly to combine ingredients and serve.

PER SERVING | Calories: 257 | Fat: 0 g | Protein: 3 g | Sodium: 19 mg | Fiber: 12 g | Carbohydrates: 66 g | Sugar: 4 g

Entrées

Grilled Flank Steak

Cilantro contains an antibacterial compound that may prove to be a safe, natural means of fighting Salmonella, a frequent cause of foodborne illness and bacterial imbalance.

INGREDIENTS | SERVES 4

½ cup coconut aminos

¼ cup Beef Stock (see recipe in Chapter 14)

3 tablespoons olive oil

⅓ cup chopped fresh cilantro

2 tablespoons chopped gingerroot

1 pound flank steak

What Are Coconut Aminos?

Coconut aminos are a soy sauce substitute made from the sap of a coconut tree. As the name implies, coconut aminos are rich in several of the amino acids, including glutamic acid, which helps digestive function. Coconut aminos are often available at your local health food store. Alternatively, you may find them near the soy sauce in your regular supermarket.

1. Mix together all ingredients except steak in a large bowl. Separate out ¼ cup of marinade and set aside. Add meat to marinade.

2. Marinate for at least 2 hours or overnight in refrigerator, turning meat occasionally.

3. Preheat grill on medium-high.

4. Grill steak for 10–15 minutes on each side, or to desired doneness; as it grills, brush with reserved marinade.

5. Let meat rest for 10 minutes. Slice meat diagonally across the grain and serve.

PER SERVING | Calories: 342 | Fat: 103 g | Protein: 31 g | Sodium: 696 mg | Fiber: 0 g | Carbohydrates: 0 g | Sugar: 0 g

Garlic Chicken Stir-Fry

Stir-fries are the perfect quick meal when you come in from a long day and want to get dinner on the table quickly.

INGREDIENTS | SERVES 4

1 tablespoon olive oil
1 cup broccoli florets
1 medium yellow onion, quartered
1 cup carrot matchsticks
1 cup snow peas
1 cup sliced button mushrooms
1 tablespoon minced garlic
4 tablespoons filtered water, divided
1 pound boneless, skinless chicken breasts, cut into 1" cubes
1 teaspoon all-natural sea salt

MSG in Take-Out

Monosodium glutamate, otherwise known as MSG, is a powerful additive and flavor enhancer. In the late 1960s and early 1970s, people started referring to the effects of MSG as Chinese Restaurant Syndrome, when people sometimes experienced headaches, tightness in the chest, feelings of weakness, and hot sensations shortly after eating takeout Chinese food. Even today, MSG is often used at restaurants, so it's much healthier to make your own stir-fries at home.

1. Heat olive oil in a large skillet or wok over medium heat.

2. Sauté broccoli, onion, carrots, snow peas, and mushrooms with garlic and 2 tablespoons water.

3. Cover skillet and cook vegetables for 3 minutes. Uncover and continue cooking vegetables for another 3 minutes, tossing constantly.

4. Add chicken and remaining water to skillet.

5. Stir-fry mixture until chicken is completely cooked through with juices running clear, about 6 minutes.

6. Sprinkle with salt, remove from heat, and enjoy.

PER SERVING | Calories: 143 | Fat: 5 g | Protein: 14 g | Sodium: 663 mg | Fiber: 3 g | Carbohydrates: 10 g | Sugar: 4 g

Coconut Shrimp

This simple recipe is a delicious and clean version of the delectable coconut shrimp we all know and love . . . and since you made it, you know what's in it!

INGREDIENTS | SERVES 2

1 cup Homemade Almond Milk (see recipe in Chapter 10)
1 cup unsweetened coconut flakes
1 tablespoon coconut oil
8 large shrimp, peeled and deveined, tail removed

1. In 2 shallow bowls, set up a dipping station with almond milk in one and coconut flakes in the other.

2. Heat coconut oil in a large skillet over medium heat.

3. Submerge shrimp in almond milk. Take shrimp, 1 at a time, out of almond milk and roll in coconut flakes to cover.

4. Place shrimp in skillet and cook for 2–3 minutes. Flip shrimp and continue cooking until shrimp are cooked through and coconut flakes are golden brown, another 2–3 minutes.

PER SERVING | Calories: 249 | Fat: 21 g | Protein: 6 g | Sodium: 44 mg | Fiber: 4 g | Carbohydrates: 12 g | Sugar: 8 g

Grilled Lemon Salmon

One 4-ounce serving of wild salmon provides a full day's requirement of vitamin D and is a good source of omega-3 fatty acids.

INGREDIENTS | SERVES 4

1½ pounds salmon fillets

⅛ teaspoon lemon pepper

1 tablespoon minced fresh rosemary or thyme

⅓ cup coconut aminos

⅓ cup fresh lemon juice

⅓ cup filtered water

½ cup extra-light olive oil

1. Cut the salmon fillet into four equal portions. Sprinkle fillets with lemon pepper and rosemary.

2. Mix together coconut aminos, lemon juice, water, and olive oil.

3. Place fish in a large resealable plastic bag with marinade mixture, seal, and turn to coat. Refrigerate for 2 hours, turning several times.

4. Lightly oil a grill or large skillet. Place salmon on cooking surface and discard marinade. Cook salmon for about 6–8 minutes per side, or until the fish flakes easily. Serve.

PER SERVING | Calories: 248 | Fat: 21 g | Protein: 6 g | Sodium: 44 mg | Fiber: 4 g | Carbohydrates: 12 g | Sugar: 8 g

Pork Loin with Baked Apples

Rather than dipping your pork in applesauce, why not build apples into the meal itself? Aromatic, tasty, and satisfying, this delicious combination of salty pork and sweet baked apples will surely become one of your favorites.

INGREDIENTS | SERVES 4

¼ cup unsweetened applesauce

2 tablespoons filtered water

3 Gala apples, peeled, cored, and sliced

1 teaspoon ground cinnamon

1 pound pork tenderloin

1 teaspoon all-natural sea salt

Homemade Olive Oil Spray

Rather than purchasing a canned aerosol olive oil spray, you can easily make your own at home. Just purchase a BPA-free plastic spray bottle (available at most grocery and hardware stores), and fill it with extra-virgin olive oil for a homemade, aerosol-free spray without chemicals or additives.

1. Preheat oven to 400°F. Grease a 9" × 13" baking pan.

2. Mix applesauce, water, and apples in a medium mixing bowl with cinnamon.

3. Layer apples evenly in prepared pan. Bake for 20 minutes, or until slightly softened.

4. Move apples aside to place pork tenderloin in the middle of the pan. Surround with apples.

5. Sprinkle tenderloin with the sea salt.

6. Return pan to oven. Bake for 30 minutes, or until internal temperature reads 165°F. Let rest for 10 minutes before slicing and serving.

PER SERVING | Calories: 204 | Fat: 3 g | Protein: 24 g | Sodium: 650 mg | Fiber: 2 g | Carbohydrates: 22 g | Sugar: 18 g

Scallops with Chives

Lots of people don't make scallops at home because they assume that they're difficult to prepare. Try this recipe to set the record straight. It's simple to make but has restaurant-quality taste.

INGREDIENTS | SERVES 2

1 pound bay scallops

1 tablespoon coconut milk

2 tablespoons chopped fresh chives

1 teaspoon all-natural sea salt

Health Benefits of Scallops

Packed with vitamin B_{12}, omega-3s, and manganese, scallops make for great cardiovascular guardians that promote optimum blood flow, prevent clots, and help maintain low blood pressure.

1. In a shallow dish, soak scallops in coconut milk for 1 hour.

2. Preheat oven to 400°F. Grease a 9" × 9" glass baking dish.

3. Place scallops in prepared baking dish. Pour coconut milk over scallops and top with chives and sea salt.

4. Bake for about 15–20 minutes, or until scallops are firm and opaque. Serve.

PER SERVING | Calories: 305 | Fat: 2 g | Protein: 48 g | Sodium: 1,772 mg | Fiber: 0 g | Carbohydrates: 12 g | Sugar: 12 g

Roast Lemon Chicken

You can add potato wedges to the pan in this recipe. Just make sure to add enough water to almost cover the potatoes, along with the juice of 1 more lemon and 2 more tablespoons of olive oil.

INGREDIENTS | SERVES 4

2 medium lemons
1 (3-pound) whole chicken
½ teaspoon sea salt
⅛ teaspoon ground black pepper
2 tablespoons extra-virgin olive oil
1 tablespoon prepared yellow mustard
1 teaspoon dried oregano

Lemons for Digestion

Lemons help trigger peristalsis—the muscular contractions that help move food along your digestive tract. Because of this, they help eliminate waste and prevent constipation.

1. Preheat oven to 400°F.

2. Cut the lemons in half and squeeze the juice into a separate container. Save the juiced lemon halves.

3. Wash chicken well inside and out and pat dry. Sprinkle inside and out with salt and pepper. Stuff squeezed-out lemon halves into cavity. Place chicken breast-side down on a rack in a shallow roasting dish. Combine lemon juice, olive oil, mustard, and oregano; brush over entire chicken.

4. Bake for 60–70 minutes, making sure to turn chicken over halfway through baking time and baste it regularly with juices from pan.

5. To test if it's done, prick with a fork and see if juices run clear, or test with meat thermometer for 165°F. When done, turn off oven and cover chicken in aluminum foil. Let rest in warm oven for 10 minutes.

6. Serve hot with pan juices.

PER SERVING | Calories: 483 | Fat: 30 g | Protein: 0 g | Sodium: 135 mg | Fiber: 0 g | Carbohydrates: 0 g | Sugar: 0 g

Pork with Leeks and Celery

Only use the white ends of the leeks and not the green stalks for this dish.

INGREDIENTS | SERVES 4

2 pounds pork shoulder
1 medium red onion, finely chopped
½ cup extra-virgin olive oil
½ cup unsweetened apple juice
2 cups filtered water
2 pounds leeks, chopped
1 cup finely chopped celery
1 cup diced tomatoes (drained if canned)
1 teaspoon dried oregano
⅛ teaspoon sea salt
⅛ teaspoon ground black pepper

The Benefits of Olive Oil

Olive oil stimulates the gallbladder to release more bile, the digestive juice that allows you to properly digest fats. The phenols in olive oil also protect the colon, reducing your risk of colon cancer.

1. Wash pork well. Chop into 1" cubes and set aside to drain on paper towels.

2. In a deep skillet, sauté onion in olive oil over medium heat until slightly soft, about 4 minutes; add pork and brown thoroughly.

3. Add apple juice to skillet. Bring to a boil, then reduce to a simmer. Cover and simmer for 15 minutes, stirring regularly. Remove pork. Cover to keep warm and set aside.

4. Add water to skillet along with leeks and celery. Bring to a boil and simmer for 30 minutes over medium heat.

5. Return pork to skillet along with tomatoes, oregano, salt, and pepper. Stir well. Bring to a boil, then reduce to a simmer and cook until sauce is reduced and thickened, approximately 8–10 minutes. Serve immediately.

PER SERVING | Calories: 997 | Fat: 71 g | Protein: 56 g | Sodium: 200 mg | Fiber: 5 g | Carbohydrates: 34 g | Sugar: 15 g

Sweet Chicken Curry

Peach preserves make this sweet, and if your dinner guests prefer less spice, you can ditch the curry, garlic, and ginger.

INGREDIENTS | SERVES 4

1 (10-ounce) package frozen green beans

1½ cups carrots, cut into matchsticks

1 tablespoon olive oil

1 medium red onion, diced

2 medium cloves garlic, minced

¼ cup raisins

1 cup Basic Chicken Stock (see recipe in Chapter 14)

⅓ cup peach preserves, no sugar added

1 tablespoon arrowroot or tapioca powder

1 tablespoon filtered water

3 cups shredded cooked chicken

2 teaspoons grated gingerroot, or 1 teaspoon ground ginger

1 teaspoon curry powder

1. Place green beans and carrots in a medium glass bowl; cover and microwave for about 6 minutes or until veggies are slightly softened. Set aside.

2. Heat olive oil on medium-high in a large skillet. Add onion, garlic, and raisins. Sauté for 5 minutes, or until onion is translucent.

3. Add chicken stock and peach preserves to skillet and bring to a boil.

4. In a small bowl, combine arrowroot or tapioca powder with water. Whisk mixture into skillet, and cook for 1 minute. Reduce heat to medium-low, add green beans, carrots, chicken, ginger, and curry powder. Heat through, about 3–5 minutes.

PER SERVING | Calories: 127 | Fat: 4 g | Protein: 5 g | Sodium: 60 mg | Fiber: 4 g | Carbohydrates: 18 g | Sugar: 13 g

Shepherd's Pie

This classic family favorite was begging for a gut-healthy makeover. This recipe's unique blend of spices and fresh ingredients give you all the comforting flavor you love without the gut-damaging ingredients you don't. Enjoy it tonight, then freeze the leftovers.

INGREDIENTS | SERVES 8

3 teaspoons olive oil

1 pound browned ground turkey breast

1 small yellow onion, minced

2 teaspoons garlic powder, divided

2 teaspoons onion powder, divided

1 teaspoon all-natural sea salt, divided

1 teaspoon ground black pepper, divided

2 cups frozen peas

2 cups cauliflower florets

1. Preheat oven to 350°F. Coat a 9" × 9" baking dish with olive oil.

2. In a mixing bowl, combine browned ground turkey breast, half of the minced onion, 1 teaspoon garlic powder, 1 teaspoon onion powder, ½ teaspoon salt, and ½ teaspoon pepper, and blend well.

3. Spread seasoned turkey meat in an even layer in bottom of prepared pan, cover with peas, and sprinkle with remaining minced onion.

4. Steam cauliflower until soft and purée in a food processor until smooth. Stir remaining spices into puréed cauliflower and spoon over peas in pan, spreading evenly.

5. Bake for 30 minutes, or until cauliflower begins to turn golden.

PER SERVING | Calories: 149 | Fat: 1 g | Protein: 17 g | Sodium: 462 mg | Fiber: 2 g | Carbohydrates: 17 g | Sugar: 2 g

Brined Grilled Chicken

Brining adds great flavor to chicken breasts and keeps them exceptionally moist.

INGREDIENTS | SERVES 6

3 tablespoons all-natural sea salt

6 cups filtered water, divided

6 small (4-ounce) bone-in, skin-on chicken breasts

2 tablespoons fresh lemon juice

4 medium cloves garlic, minced

2 medium shallots, minced

1 teaspoon dried oregano

¼ teaspoon ground cayenne pepper

3 tablespoons tomato paste

2 tablespoons olive oil

Brining Chicken

Don't go overboard on the salt when brining, as too much salt can result in the outer layer of flesh becoming salty and tough. Brine for only the recommended time, and do not rinse the chicken after brining.

1. In a medium bowl, combine salt and 1 cup water, stirring to dissolve. Add 2 more cups water and mix.

2. Place chicken breasts, skin-side down, in a large glass baking dish. Pour brine over chicken breasts; add remaining 3 cups water. Cover and refrigerate for 3–4 hours.

3. When ready to cook, preheat grill on medium. In a small bowl, combine remaining ingredients and mix well. Remove chicken from brine; discard brine. Loosen skin from chicken breasts and rub half of the garlic mixture onto the flesh. Smooth skin back over chicken.

4. Rub remaining garlic mixture over chicken skin. Let stand for 15 minutes. Place skin-side down on grill, 6" from heat. Cover and grill for 8 minutes, then turn. Cover and grill 8 minutes longer, then check chicken for doneness. Grill until meat is no longer pink or until a meat thermometer reads 165°F.

PER SERVING | Calories: 156 | Fat: 4 g | Protein: 36 g | Sodium: 365 mg | Fiber: 0 g | Carbohydrates: 1 g | Sugar: 1 g

Asian Steaks

Asian flavors infuse this tender steak. Serve it with a napa cabbage salad and fresh fruit for dessert.

INGREDIENTS | SERVES 4

1 tablespoon minced gingerroot

2 medium cloves garlic, minced

1 medium shallot, minced

½ teaspoon five spice powder

2 tablespoons rice wine vinegar

1 tablespoon fresh lime juice

2 teaspoons coconut aminos

2 tablespoons olive oil

⅛ teaspoon ground cayenne pepper

1 pound flank steak

Cutting Steaks

When cutting steaks after they are cooked, you have to wait. If steaks are cut into right off the grill or griddle, the juice will run all over your serving plate. Let the steaks stand, covered, for 5–10 minutes to allow the juices to redistribute. Then serve or slice the meat.

1. In a large resealable plastic bag, combine all ingredients except flank steak. Add steak, seal bag, and knead bag gently to coat meat.

2. Place bag in a large pan and refrigerate overnight, turning the bag occasionally.

3. When ready to eat, prepare and preheat grill on medium. Remove steak from marinade; discard marinade.

4. Grill steak 6" from heat for 12–16 minutes or to desired doneness, turning once. Cover with foil and let stand for 5 minutes. Slice across the grain to serve.

PER SERVING | Calories: 282 | Fat: 16 g | Protein: 31 g | Sodium: 62 mg | Fiber: 0 g | Carbohydrates: 3 g | Sugar: 0 g

Stovetop Fish

You can choose any whitefish you want for this recipe. Halibut, striped bass, and haddock all have a mild taste that takes goes well with garlic, tomatoes, and mint.

INGREDIENTS | SERVES 4

2 pounds whitefish fillets

3 tablespoons extra-virgin olive oil

4 medium cloves garlic, minced

1 pound ripe tomatoes, peeled and minced

6 fresh mint leaves, finely chopped

⅛ teaspoon sea salt

⅛ teaspoon ground black pepper

1 tablespoon dried oregano

½ cup filtered water

1 small bunch fresh flat-leaf parsley, chopped

Roast Tomatoes for Easy Peeling

Roasting tomatoes not only makes it easy to peel their skin off, but it also gives the tomato a nice, smoked flavor that enhances your dish. Turn your broiler on and position a rack about 6" from the heat. Remove the tomato stems, cut the tomatoes in half, and place them cut-side down on a rimmed baking sheet. Let the tomatoes broil until their skins are slightly blackened. Remove the tomatoes from the oven and allow them to cool. Once cool enough to handle, you should be able to pull the skin right off.

1. Wash fish fillets and pat dry with paper towels.

2. Heat olive oil in a large frying pan on medium and sauté garlic for 30 seconds.

3. Add tomatoes, mint, salt, pepper, and oregano. Bring to a boil, then reduce to a simmer. Simmer for 10 minutes, until thickened.

4. Add water and continue to simmer for another 3–4 minutes.

5. Place fish in pan and allow to simmer for 15 minutes. Do not stir; simply shake the pan gently from time to time to avoid sticking.

6. Garnish with chopped parsley and serve immediately.

PER SERVING | Calories: 261 | Fat: 12 g | Protein: 33 g | Sodium: 122 mg | Fiber: 1 g | Carbohydrates: 5 g | Sugar: 4 g

Skillet Chops and Veggies

This easy one-dish meal is pure comfort food. Serve with a butter lettuce salad mixed with mushrooms and green bell peppers.

INGREDIENTS | SERVES 4

4 small (4-ounce) boneless loin pork chops

2 tablespoons almond flour

½ teaspoon all-natural sea salt

⅛ teaspoon ground black pepper

2 tablespoons olive oil

1 medium yellow onion, chopped

3 medium cloves garlic, minced

4 medium russet potatoes, peeled and thinly sliced

3 medium carrots, peeled and sliced

1 cup Basic Chicken Stock (see recipe in Chapter 14)

1 tablespoon fresh lemon juice

1. Sprinkle chops with flour, salt, and pepper. In a large, deep skillet, heat olive oil over medium heat. Add chops and brown for 2–3 minutes on each side. Remove chops from pan and set aside.

2. Add onion and garlic to skillet; cook and stir until crisp-tender, about 5 minutes.

3. Add potatoes to pan; cook and stir until potatoes are coated. Top with carrots, then add browned pork chops.

4. Add chicken stock and lemon juice and bring to a simmer. Cover skillet tightly, reduce heat to medium-low, and simmer for 35–45 minutes, or until potatoes are tender and chops are cooked, shaking pan occasionally. Serve immediately.

PER SERVING | Calories: 413 | Fat: 16 g | Protein: 25 g | Sodium: 1,026 mg | Fiber: 7 g | Carbohydrates: 43 g | Sugar: 8 g

Thai Vegetable Curry

The background of light nutty sweetness from the almond butter gives these fresh vegetables a nice flavor that's accented beautifully with the curry powder and garlic.

INGREDIENTS | SERVES 2

1 medium eggplant, chopped

1 medium zucchini, chopped

1 tablespoon olive oil

1 cup coconut milk, divided

3 tablespoons almond butter

1 teaspoon minced garlic

1 medium yellow onion, minced

2 medium stalks celery, minced

2 teaspoons curry powder

1. In a large skillet, sauté eggplant and zucchini in olive oil over medium heat until softened, about 8–10 minutes.

2. Add ½ cup coconut milk, almond butter, garlic, onion, celery, and curry powder and bring to a simmer.

3. Add remaining coconut milk as a thinner if needed, and remove from heat. Serve hot.

PER SERVING | Calories: 500 | Fat: 38 g | Protein: 9 g | Sodium: 66 mg | Fiber: 14 g | Carbohydrates: 40 g | Sugar: 20 g

Grilled Jumbo Shrimp

To devein shrimp, use a paring knife and cut a ¼"-deep slit along the shrimp's back. You will see a black or white "vein." Use the point of your knife to lift the vein and gently pull the vein back to remove it.

INGREDIENTS | SERVES 4

2 pounds jumbo shrimp, deveined but unpeeled

¼ cup extra-virgin olive oil

Juice of 1 medium lemon

4 medium cloves garlic, minced

1 tablespoon lemon zest

⅛ teaspoon sea salt

⅛ teaspoon ground black pepper

2 tablespoons light olive oil, divided

1. Wash shrimp well under running water and set aside to drain.

2. In a medium mixing bowl, combine extra-virgin olive oil, lemon juice, garlic, lemon zest, salt, and pepper.

3. Add shrimp to marinade and toss well. Marinate in refrigerator for 2 hours, periodically tossing shrimp in marinade.

4. Lightly coat grill with 1 tablespoon light olive oil and preheat on medium. Butterfly shrimp lengthwise just below the head and spread open. Brush shrimp liberally with remaining marinade.

5. Grill shrimp shell-side down for 1 minute. Turn shrimp and grill until lightly browned, about 1 minute. Turn shrimp over again, brush liberally with remaining olive oil, and grill for about 1 minute longer. Remove and serve immediately.

PER SERVING | Calories: 353 | Fat: 23 g | Protein: 34 g | Sodium: 311 mg | Fiber: 0 g | Carbohydrates: 0 g | Sugar: 0 g

Aegean Baked Sole

You can use turbot, halibut, or flounder as substitutes for the sole in this recipe.

INGREDIENTS | SERVES 4

1½ pounds sole fillets

½ teaspoon sea salt

⅛ teaspoon ground black pepper

2 medium lemons

4 tablespoons extra-virgin olive oil, divided

1 teaspoon dried oregano

¼ cup capers, rinsed

¼ cup chopped fresh dill

2 tablespoons chopped green onion (or celery leaves or parsley)

1. Preheat oven to 350°F.

2. Wash fish well under cold water and pat dry with paper towels. Sprinkle fish with salt and pepper and set aside.

3. Slice 1 lemon into thin slices, then cut slices in half.

4. Pour 2 tablespoons olive oil into a 9" x 13" baking dish; layer fish and lemon slices alternately.

5. Sprinkle oregano, capers, dill, and green onion over fish and lemon slices.

6. Drizzle remaining olive oil and squeeze juice of remaining lemon over everything.

7. Cover and bake for 30 minutes.

PER SERVING | Calories: 339 | Fat: 17 g | Protein: 42 g | Sodium: 675 mg | Fiber: 2 g | Carbohydrates: 5 g | Sugar: 1 g

Grilled Salmon with Dill

Salmon is marinated for a while, then grilled to perfection in this delicious and easy recipe. Serve with roasted potatoes and steamed veggies.

INGREDIENTS | SERVES 4

¼ cup unsweetened orange juice
1 tablespoon fresh lemon juice
2 tablespoons olive oil
1 tablespoon Dijon mustard
2 medium cloves garlic, minced
½ teaspoon dried dill weed
4 (6-ounce) salmon steaks
1 tablespoon olive oil for oiling grill

Salmon

Salmon is an essential part of a healthy diet. If you can, try to eat it twice a week. It contains omega-3 fatty acids, which are essential nutrients that your body cannot make. The fats in salmon help lower the risk of heart disease, reduce cholesterol levels, and reduce blood-clotting ability, which can help prevent heart attacks.

1. In a 9" × 13" glass dish, combine orange juice, lemon juice, olive oil, mustard, garlic, and dill. Add salmon steaks; turn to coat. Cover and refrigerate for 1–2 hours.

2. Preheat grill. Make sure grill is clean. Lightly oil grill rack with olive oil. Remove salmon from marinade and discard marinade.

3. Grill salmon 6" from heat for 9–12 minutes or until fish flakes easily with a fork, turning once.

PER SERVING | Calories: 328 | Fat: 21 g | Protein: 33 g | Sodium: 121 mg | Fiber: 0 g | Carbohydrates: 2 g | Sugar: 1 g

CHAPTER 12

Sides

Roasted Eggplant

Large eggplants are the best for this recipe, but you can use smaller ones, too.

INGREDIENTS | SERVES 4

2 large eggplants

¼ cup minced fresh herbs, such as rosemary, thyme, oregano

1 tablespoon minced garlic

1 tablespoon extra-virgin olive oil

2 tablespoons sesame seeds

1. Preheat oven to 350°F.

2. Slice eggplants in half, lengthwise. Make deep cuts with a small knife diagonally across the flesh, from left to right horizontally, and then vertically. Do not cut through the skin.

3. Fill all cuts in eggplants with herbs and garlic.

4. Place eggplants skin-side down in a large ovenproof dish and drizzle with olive oil.

5. Bake until soft and slightly brown, about 45 minutes. Check eggplant during baking and cover dish with aluminum foil if needed to prevent eggplant from overbrowning.

6. Sprinkle sesame seeds over eggplant and cook for 2 more minutes.

PER SERVING | Calories: 139 | Fat: 7 g | Protein: 4 g | Sodium: 8 mg | Fiber: 12 g | Carbohydrates: 20 g | Sugar: 8 g

Seasoned Oven Fries

Since fast-food fries are out of the question, try a healthier version. This recipe also works well with sweet potatoes, although you may want to experiment with the seasonings if you go that route.

INGREDIENTS | SERVES 4

2 large Yukon gold potatoes, peeled and cut into wedges

2 tablespoons extra-virgin olive oil

¼ teaspoon all-natural sea salt

¼ teaspoon dried thyme (optional)

1. Preheat oven to 450°F.

2. Toss potato wedges with oil, salt, and thyme (if using).

3. Spread out potatoes on a rimmed baking sheet.

4. Bake until browned and tender, turning once, about 30 minutes. Serve.

PER SERVING | Calories: 180 | Fat: 10 g | Protein: 15 g | Sodium: 649 mg | Fiber: 1 g | Carbohydrates: 8 g | Sugar: 2 g

Scrumptious Sage and Squash Soup

Combining the sweet scrumptiousness of squash with aromatic and tasty sage, this soup is a surefire hit. Completely void of the poor ingredients that most canned soup varieties would include, this is a homemade delight you can enjoy anytime.

INGREDIENTS | SERVES 4

1 pound summer squash (about 3 cups cubed)

4 cups filtered water

2 teaspoons all-natural sea salt

½ cup dried sage (plus extra for garnish: optional)

Brighten Flavors with Spices

Many herbs are actually more powerful in their dried versions, so if you substitute dried herbs for fresh herbs, make sure to adjust measurements accordingly. For a stronger taste in soups, opt for dried spices . . . unless it's a garnish.

1. Peel squash and remove seeds. Cut into 1" cubes. Set aside.

2. Bring water to a boil in a large pot over medium heat.

3. Reduce heat to low, add squash, salt, and sage. Simmer for about 20–25 minutes, or until fork-tender.

4. Using an immersion blender, emulsify the squash and sage until smooth.

5. Serve hot or cold, and garnish with extra crumbled sage leaves if desired.

PER SERVING | Calories: 26 | Fat: 1 g | Protein: 1 g | Sodium: 1,188 mg | Fiber: 3 g | Carbohydrates: 5 g | Sugar: 2 g

Zucchini Fritters

You do not need to peel the zucchini, but you must peel the potato for use in this recipe.

INGREDIENTS | SERVES 4

2 large eggs
2 tablespoons finely chopped fresh mint
1 tablespoon dried oregano
1 large clove garlic, minced
1 tablespoon extra-virgin olive oil
2 tablespoons almond meal (or more as needed)
½ teaspoon sea salt
⅛ teaspoon ground black pepper
½ teaspoon baking powder
1 tablespoon olive oil for frying
1 medium zucchini
1 medium white potato, peeled
½ medium white onion

1. In a small bowl, beat eggs well. Add mint, oregano, garlic, extra-virgin olive oil, almond meal, salt, pepper, and baking powder. Mix well to achieve a thick batter-like consistency. If the mixture is thin, add more almond meal to thicken slightly.

2. Add olive oil to a 10" skillet (depth of oil should be no more than ½"). Heat on medium for about 3–4 minutes, until thoroughly heated.

3. Meanwhile, wash zucchini and potato; shred into a large mixing bowl using a grater or shredder. Mince onion; add to bowl. Stir batter into zucchini mixture.

4. Using a large spoon, add portions of zucchini mixture to hot oil in clumps, making sure to form them as small pancakes. Work quickly so mixture does not become watery. (Zucchini will begin to seep water immediately upon shredding.)

5. Cook about 3–4 minutes. Carefully turn fritters with a small spatula or large fork and cook for another 3–4 minutes, until golden brown.

6. Remove from pan and drain on paper towels. Serve hot.

PER SERVING | Calories: 174 | Fat: 11 g | Protein: 6 g | Sodium: 279 mg | Fiber: 3 g | Carbohydrates: 15 g | Sugar: 2 g

Roasted Brussels Sprouts

Coconut oil and balsamic vinegar add a little zing to Brussels sprouts.
Try serving with mashed cauliflower and chicken or fish.

INGREDIENTS | SERVES 6

1 pound Brussels sprouts

2 tablespoons melted coconut oil

2 tablespoons balsamic vinegar, no sulfites added

½ teaspoon all-natural sea salt

⅛ teaspoon ground black pepper

1. Preheat oven to 375°F. Grease a baking sheet.

2. Peel off tough outer layer of Brussels sprouts and slice each sprout in half. Place sprouts on prepared baking sheet.

3. In a small bowl, mix together melted coconut oil and vinegar. Using a basting brush, coat Brussels sprouts evenly with oil mixture. Sprinkle with salt and pepper.

4. Roast sprouts for 10 minutes. Turn and roast for another 10 minutes, or until lightly browned and easily pierced with a fork. Remove from oven and serve.

PER SERVING | Calories: 76 | Fat: 5 g | Protein: 3 g | Sodium: 20 mg | Fiber: 3 g | Carbohydrates: 8 g | Sugar: 2 g

Roasted Beets

It's a good idea to wear kitchen gloves when preparing this recipe, since beet juice can stain the skin.

INGREDIENTS | SERVES 4

6 medium beets
3 medium sweet potatoes
2 large carrots
2½ tablespoons olive oil, divided
1 teaspoon garlic powder
1 teaspoon all-natural sea salt
1 teaspoon ground black pepper

1. Preheat oven to 400°F.

2. Wash beets, sweet potatoes, and carrots. Peel sweet potatoes and carrots and cut all into chunks.

3. In a large bowl, toss the beets with ½ tablespoon olive oil to coat.

4. Spread in a single layer on a baking sheet. Bake beets for 15 minutes.

5. Meanwhile, mix together remaining 2 tablespoons olive oil, garlic powder, salt, and pepper in a large resealable plastic bag. Add sweet potatoes and carrots. Seal and shake to coat vegetables with oil mixture.

6. Remove beets from oven. Mix sweet potato and carrot mixture with beets on baking sheet. Bake for 45 minutes, stirring after 20 minutes, until all vegetables are tender. Serve.

PER SERVING | Calories: 291 | Fat: 9 g | Protein: 5 g | Sodium: 151 mg | Fiber: 9 g | Carbohydrates: 50 g | Sugar: 14 g

Lemon Root Vegetables

You might not have cooked with parsnips before, but they resemble pale carrots and the flavor is slightly stronger. You can substitute them for carrots in many recipes.

INGREDIENTS | SERVES 4

4 medium carrots
2 medium rutabagas (about 2 cups)
2 medium parsnips (about 1 cup)
½ cup filtered water
2 tablespoons olive oil
1 tablespoon unsweetened apple juice concentrate
1 tablespoon fresh lemon juice
½ teaspoon lemon zest
½ teaspoon dried parsley flakes

1. Peel and cut vegetables into 3" julienne strips.

2. In a large saucepan, combine the carrots, rutabaga, parsnips, and water. Bring to a boil. Reduce heat to medium; cover and cook for about 15 minutes, until fork-tender.

3. In a small saucepan, combine remaining ingredients; cook, uncovered, over medium heat for 2—3 minutes.

4. Drain vegetables; add olive oil mixture. Cook for 3–4 minutes or until vegetables are glazed, stirring occasionally.

PER SERVING | Calories: 136 | Fat: 7 g | Protein: 2 g | Sodium: 60 mg | Fiber: 5 g | Carbohydrates: 18 g | Sugar: 9 g

Mashed Sweet Potatoes

You don't have to prepare sweet potatoes with crunchy or candy toppings to make them delicious. This is a tasty, and very nutritious, alternative to the traditional serving of buttered mashed potatoes. If you like sweet potatoes, you'll love this side.

INGREDIENTS | SERVES 8

3 large sweet potatoes, peeled and cubed

1 teaspoon ground cinnamon

1 teaspoon ground nutmeg

1 cup Homemade Almond Milk (see recipe in Chapter 10)

Getting Creative

You can get creative with mashed sweet potatoes by using them as a base in your next Shepherd's Pie (see Chapter 11) instead of the mashed cauliflower. If you're really looking for a treat, layer mashed sweet potatoes over the mashed cauliflower.

1. Place sweet potatoes in a large saucepan. Add enough water to cover potatoes. Bring to a boil over medium heat. Reduce heat to low, and simmer until fork-tender, about 30 minutes.

2. Remove potatoes from heat, drain, and return to saucepan.

3. Add cinnamon and nutmeg to sweet potatoes. Mash or beat until smooth, adding almond milk ¼ cup at a time until desired consistency is reached.

4. Serve hot.

PER SERVING | Calories: 71 | Fat: 0 g | Protein: 1 g | Sodium: 44 mg | Fiber: 2 g | Carbohydrates: 16 g | Sugar: 8 g

Caramelized Spiced Carrots

This is a simple side dish that is full of flavor. Serve it with grilled or roasted chicken, or during the holidays along with a baked ham.

INGREDIENTS | SERVES 4

1¼ pounds baby carrots

¼ cup unsweetened orange juice

⅛ teaspoon all-natural sea salt

⅛ teaspoon ground white pepper

1 teaspoon orange zest

1 tablespoon grated gingerroot

1 tablespoon olive oil

Baby Carrots

Since appearing on the market not so very long ago, baby carrots have overtaken regular carrots in sales. They are not technically baby carrots, but a carrot variety called Imperator that is grown to be longer and sweeter than regular carrots. The carrots are then trimmed down to the characteristic size and shape of baby carrots.

1. In a large saucepan, combine carrots, orange juice, salt, and pepper. Bring to a boil over high heat, then reduce heat to low, cover, and cook for 3–4 minutes, or until carrots are crisp-tender.

2. Add orange zest, gingerroot, and olive oil, and bring to a boil over high heat. Cook until most of the orange juice evaporates and the carrots start to brown, stirring frequently, about 4–5 minutes. Serve immediately.

PER SERVING | Calories: 92 | Fat: 4 g | Protein: 1 g | Sodium: 189 mg | Fiber: 4 g | Carbohydrates: 14 g | Sugar: 8 g

Briami (Baked Vegetable Medley)

Feel free to add radishes, sweet potatoes, or any other vegetable that strikes your fancy to add more variety to this dish.

INGREDIENTS | SERVES 4

2 large eggplants, cubed

2 medium zucchini, cubed

2 large red potatoes, cubed

2 large parsnips, peeled and thickly sliced

2 large carrots, peeled and thickly sliced

1 pound button mushrooms, thickly sliced

1 large yellow onion, sliced

1 large red bell pepper, cut into strips

6 medium cloves garlic, cut in half

½ cup extra-virgin olive oil

1 tablespoon finely chopped fresh rosemary

½ tablespoon dried oregano

½ teaspoon sea salt

⅛ teaspoon ground black pepper

1. Preheat oven to 400°F.

2. Place cubed eggplant in a colander and sprinkle with salt. Place colander over a plate and let stand for 30 minutes to drain bitter juices.

3. Rinse eggplant and combine all vegetables and garlic in a large baking dish. Add olive oil and mix well. Sprinkle with rosemary, oregano, salt, and pepper. Add enough water to cover vegetables.

4. Bake uncovered for 50–60 minutes, or until water has been absorbed. Make sure to stir vegetables at least once halfway through cooking time, or as needed. Serve warm.

PER SERVING | Calories: 548 | Fat: 27 g | Protein: 13 g | Sodium: 297 mg | Fiber: 21 g | Carbohydrates: 74 g | Sugar: 21 g

Make It a Meal

You can make this a complete meal by browning some ground beef, chicken, or turkey in a skillet and then adding it to the mixture before it goes into the oven.

Dandelion Greens

Be sure to wash these greens well and cut away all of the root stalk when cleaning, as it is tough and does not become tender when cooked. This dish makes a great side with grilled fish.

INGREDIENTS | SERVES 6

4 pounds dandelion greens
½ cup extra-virgin olive oil
½ cup fresh lemon juice
½ teaspoon sea salt
⅛ teaspoon ground black pepper

1. Cut away and discard stalks of dandelion greens; wash thoroughly.

2. Bring a large pot of water to a rolling boil; add greens and stir. Cook over high heat until greens are tender, about 8–10 minutes; remove and drain well.

3. Combine olive oil, lemon juice, salt, and pepper; use as a dressing for greens.

4. Serve warm or cold.

PER SERVING | Calories: 285 | Fat: 19 g | Protein: 8 g | Sodium: 390 mg | Fiber: 11 g | Carbohydrates: 28 g | Sugar: 3 g

Veggie Stir-Fry

Mushrooms are a good source of the antioxidant mineral selenium, which may offer some protection from prostate cancer. If you use carrots in this recipe, be sure to cut them into very small pieces to ensure that they are tender after the short cooking time.

INGREDIENTS | SERVES 4

2 tablespoons olive oil or coconut oil

3 medium cloves garlic, minced

1 small bunch green onions, thinly sliced

1 tablespoon finely sliced gingerroot

4 cups mixed vegetables: sliced mushrooms, diced carrots, broccoli florets, and snow peas (or mixed seasonal vegetables of choice)

½ cup filtered water

3 tablespoons coconut aminos

1. Heat oil in a wok or large sauté pan on medium-high heat. Add garlic, green onions, and ginger; sauté until fragrant, about 30 seconds.

2. Stir in vegetables, water, and coconut aminos.

3. Let simmer for about 5 minutes or until vegetables are crisp-tender, stirring lightly.

4. Serve warm.

PER SERVING | Calories: 113 | Fat: 7 g | Protein: 3 g | Sodium: 115 mg | Fiber: 3 g | Carbohydrates: 11 g | Sugar: 4 g

Braised Green Beans

Try using a bean slicer to remove the bean strings and cut the beans lengthwise.

INGREDIENTS | SERVES 4

½ cup extra-virgin olive oil

1 medium yellow onion, finely chopped

2 pounds fresh green beans, trimmed

1 large or 2 medium red potatoes, cut into eighths

1½ cups fresh tomato juice, sauce, or strained tomato pulp

¼ cup chopped fresh mint

½ teaspoon sea salt

⅛ teaspoon ground black pepper

1 cup filtered water

1. Heat olive oil in a large pot over medium-high heat; reduce heat to medium and sauté onion until slightly softened and translucent.

2. Add beans to pot; stir well to mix with olive oil and onion. Cover and let simmer for 10 minutes.

3. Uncover and stir. Add potatoes, tomato juice, mint, salt, pepper, and water. Stir well.

4. Bring to a boil. Reduce heat to medium-low and partially cover pot, leaving it slightly open to allow steam to escape so sauce can reduce. Let simmer for 45–60 minutes, or until beans and potatoes are tender enough to cut with fork. Stir occasionally.

PER SERVING | Calories: 381 | Fat: 26 g | Protein: 7 g | Sodium: 500 mg | Fiber: 11 g | Carbohydrates: 38 g | Sugar: 9 g

Sautéed Peas

Baby peas are tender and sweet. The savory flavors of shallots and fresh garlic complement the peas' sweet flavor nicely.

INGREDIENTS | SERVES 6

1 tablespoon olive oil

2 medium shallots, minced

3 medium cloves garlic, minced

1 (16-ounce) bag frozen peas

2 tablespoons Basic Vegetable Stock (see recipe in Chapter 14)

½ teaspoon all-natural sea salt

⅛ teaspoon ground black pepper

½ teaspoon dried thyme

1. In a large skillet, heat olive oil on medium. Add shallots and garlic; cook and stir until shallots are crisp-tender, about 4 minutes. Add remaining ingredients and bring to a simmer.

2. Cover skillet and cook, stirring occasionally, until peas are hot and tender, about 8–11 minutes. Serve immediately.

PER SERVING | Calories: 89 | Fat: 3 g | Protein: 4 g | Sodium: 250 mg | Fiber: 4 g | Carbohydrates: 13 g | Sugar: 4 g

Go Frozen

Frozen vegetables may be more nutrient-rich than fresh ones. Frozen vegetables are often processed right after picking, which preserves their nutrient content. Fresh vegetables start to lose nutrients as soon as they're picked and the longer they sit on your grocery store shelves, the more nutrients they lose.

Lemon Potatoes

Yukon gold potatoes are preferable when preparing this recipe.

INGREDIENTS | SERVES 4

2½ pounds Yukon gold potatoes, peeled
½ cup extra-virgin olive oil, divided
½ teaspoon sea salt
⅛ teaspoon ground black pepper
Juice of 2 medium lemons
1 tablespoon lemon zest
1 heaping tablespoon dried oregano

1. Preheat oven to 375°F. Cut potatoes into thin wedges slightly bigger than fries but not too big, as you want them to cook through and crisp slightly on the outside.

2. Coat the bottom and sides of a deep medium-sized baking dish with 1 tablespoon olive oil (stone bakeware works best).

3. Spread potato slices evenly across bottom of pan; sprinkle with salt and pepper.

4. Add enough water to almost, but not quite, cover bottom layer of potatoes. Add lemon juice and zest; using your hands, mix potatoes well in pan to ensure an even soaking and to distribute salt, pepper, and lemon zest.

5. Pour remaining olive oil over top of potatoes, making sure to cover all of them; sprinkle oregano over everything. Bake about 50 minutes, until edges of potatoes are visibly crisp; mix potatoes well halfway through cooking to ensure thorough and even baking.

PER SERVING | Calories: 293 | Fat: 18 g | Protein: 4 g | Sodium: 12 mg | Fiber: 4 g | Carbohydrates: 31 g | Sugar: 2 g

Sautéed Yellow Squash and Carrots

When your plate is filled with colorful veggies, you know you're maximizing your nutrient intake. This side dish is a good example of a colorful recipe.

INGREDIENTS | SERVES 6

2 tablespoons olive oil

2 medium shallots, minced

2 medium carrots, peeled and sliced

¼ cup filtered water

3 medium yellow summer squash, sliced

½ teaspoon all-natural sea salt

⅛ teaspoon ground white pepper

½ teaspoon dried sage

1. In large saucepan, heat olive oil on medium. Add shallots; cook and stir for 2 minutes. Add carrots; cook and stir for 2 minutes. Add water and bring to a simmer. Cover saucepan; simmer for 3 minutes.

2. Stir in squash and increase heat to medium-high. Simmer until liquid evaporates, stirring occasionally.

3. Stir in salt, pepper, and sage; cover and remove from heat. Let stand for 3 minutes. Stir and serve.

PER SERVING | Calories: 72 | Fat: 5 g | Protein: 2 g | Sodium: 218 mg | Fiber: 2 g | Carbohydrates: 7 g | Sugar 3 g

Summer Squash

There are two basic kinds of squash: summer and winter. Summer squash are thin-skinned and tender, cook quickly, and can be served raw. They include yellow squash and zucchini. Winter squash include pumpkins, butternut squash, and acorn squash. They are hard, with thick shells, and they must be cooked before eating.

Roasted Veggie Toss

For this recipe, you'll just chop the ingredients and throw them in a dish to bake! Besides smelling and tasting amazing, these beautiful vegetables make for a meal full of great health benefits that will also fill you up.

INGREDIENTS | SERVES 4

4 medium Idaho potatoes, cut into ½" cubes

4 large carrots, peeled and cut into ½" cubes

2 medium yellow onions, cut into ½" dice

2 tablespoons olive oil

1 teaspoon garlic powder

1 teaspoon onion powder

1 teaspoon ground turmeric

1 teaspoon dried Italian seasoning

1. Preheat oven to 400°F. Grease a 9" × 13" baking dish.

2. In a large resealable plastic bag, combine potatoes, carrots, onions, olive oil, and spices; toss to coat.

3. Pour vegetables into prepared baking dish.

4. Bake for 1 hour, stirring vegetables around at 30 minutes, and again at 45 minutes. Serve warm.

PER SERVING | Calories: 286 | Fat: 7 g | Protein: 6 g | Sodium: 64 mg | Fiber: 6 g | Carbohydrates: 53 g | Sugar: 7 g

Roasting for Powerful Flavor

Roasting vegetables can make for an incredibly different experience than sautéing or baking. By tossing vegetables in olive oil, roasting them at high heat, and flavoring them with delicious spices, you can create a crispy and satisfying variation of the vegetables you already know and love. Potatoes and carrots aren't the only ones great for roasting, either: zucchini, squash, tomatoes, onions, and celery are also great options.

Spicy Broccolini

Not too many people think of broccolini as a go-to veggie, but this is one healthy little morsel that deserves attention. This simple side dish can accent all types of meals like chicken, fish, meat, or vegetarian dishes.

INGREDIENTS | SERVES 2

1 tablespoon olive oil

1 tablespoon chopped garlic

1 pound broccolini

1 teaspoon all-natural sea salt

1 teaspoon red pepper flakes

What Is Broccolini?

Most people have heard of broccoli and many eat it on a somewhat regular basis, but broccolini is a new concept to most. A hybrid of broccoli and a Chinese variety of kale, broccolini is a delicious vegetable that many eat raw. You can find this gorgeous, long-stemmed vegetable in your grocer's fresh vegetable section and at many produce stands. They require very little time or effort to prepare into a beautiful, unique twist on the broccoli norm.

1. Heat olive oil in a large skillet over medium heat. Add garlic and sauté for 1 minute.

2. Add broccolini, salt, and red pepper flakes. Sauté for 3–5 minutes, until broccolini is crisp-tender. Serve warm.

PER SERVING | Calories: 145 | Fat: 8 g | Protein: 7 g | Sodium: 1,254 mg | Fiber: 6 g | Carbohydrates: 17 g | Sugar: 4 g

Arakas (Stewed Green Peas)

Frozen peas are an excellent choice for this dish, as they do not require shelling and are ready to go.

INGREDIENTS | SERVES 4

2 pounds shelled green peas (fresh or frozen)

½ cup extra-virgin olive oil

2 medium yellow onions, diced

3–3½ pounds potatoes, cut into chunks

1 cup diced tomatoes (drained if canned)

½ cup finely chopped fresh dill

1 teaspoon dried oregano

½ teaspoon all-natural sea salt

⅛ teaspoon ground black pepper

1 cup filtered water

1. Rinse peas in a colander and drain well.

2. Heat oil in a large skillet on medium-high and sauté onions until they begin to soften; add peas and potatoes and continue to sauté for another 3–4 minutes, stirring constantly.

3. Add tomatoes, dill, oregano, salt, pepper, and water; stir and bring to a boil. Reduce heat to medium-low and cover. Simmer for about 1 hour, until peas and potatoes are tender. Serve hot or cold.

PER SERVING | Calories: 446 | Fat: 27 g | Protein: 14 g | Sodium: 26 mg | Fiber: 14 g | Carbohydrates: 43 g | Sugar: 16 g

Perfect Acorn Squash Cups

These tender and delicious acorn squash "cups" provide perfectly portioned individual servings. These vibrant squash cups not only look and taste great, they are brimming with nutrients.

INGREDIENTS | SERVES 2

1 large acorn squash
1 tablespoon olive oil
1 teaspoon ground cinnamon
1 teaspoon all-natural sea salt

1. Preheat oven to 375°F.

2. Cut squash in half and remove seeds and pulp. Place in a roasting pan with hollowed insides facing up. Coat cut top edges and insides of squash halves with olive oil. Sprinkle cinnamon and salt on top edges and insides.

3. Bake for 30–45 minutes, or until squash flesh is fork-tender. Serve warm.

PER SERVING | Calories: 149 | Fat: 7 g | Protein: 2 g | Sodium: 1,167 mg | Fiber: 4 g | Carbohydrates: 23 g | Sugar: 0 g

CHAPTER 13

Salads and Dressings

Banana Berry Salad

This is a great salad to share at a potluck or picnic.

INGREDIENTS | SERVES 6

4 cups sliced banana
3 cups sliced strawberries
3 cups sliced kiwifruit
1 cup unsweetened coconut flakes

1. Combine banana, strawberries, and kiwifruit in a large bowl.

2. Sprinkle coconut flakes on top. Stir well to evenly coat fruit with coconut flakes.

PER SERVING | Calories: 295 | Fat: 9 g | Protein: 3 g | Sodium: 2 mg | Fiber: 11 g | Carbohydrates: 52 g | Sugar: 28 g

Asparagus Spears and Grape Tomato Toss

Blanched asparagus spears add a beautiful bright green to this delicious toss, while the grape tomatoes contribute a deep red. It's a feast for your eyes and your taste buds.

INGREDIENTS | SERVES 2

4 cups asparagus pieces (about 1" long)

2 cups halved grape tomatoes

2 tablespoons balsamic vinegar, no sulfites added

1 tablespoon extra-virgin olive oil

Choose Your Type

Green asparagus is the most common type, but the vegetable is also available in white and purple varieties. The white variety is more delicate, while the purple is lighter and fruitier in flavor. You can use any of the three for this dish.

1. In a large pot of boiling water over medium heat, blanche asparagus until bright green and still crisp, about 30–45 seconds. Remove from heat and shock with cold water to stop the cooking process.

2. Drain asparagus and place in a large mixing bowl.

3. Add tomatoes to bowl and drizzle with balsamic vinegar and olive oil. Toss to coat evenly.

PER SERVING | Calories: 154 | Fat: 7 g | Protein: 7 g | Sodium: 17 mg | Fiber: 7 g | Carbohydrates: 19 g | Sugar: 11 g

Tuna-Topped Salad

This delicious tuna recipe makes for a great standalone dish, so just imagine how tasty it is served atop crisp romaine lettuce. This is a simple dish you can be proud to serve to family or friends.

INGREDIENTS | SERVES 2

1 teaspoon coconut aminos

1 tablespoon minced garlic

2 tablespoons minced gingerroot, divided

2 tablespoons rice wine vinegar, divided

2 (4-ounce) tuna steaks

1 tablespoon olive oil

3 cups chopped romaine lettuce

1 tablespoon sesame oil

½ cup chopped green onions

1. In a shallow dish, combine coconut aminos, garlic, 1 tablespoon ginger, and 1 tablespoon vinegar. Place tuna steaks in marinade. Cover and refrigerate for 30 minutes, turning once after 15 minutes.

2. Heat olive oil in a large skillet over medium heat. Sear the tuna steaks on high heat for about 1 to 2 minutes per side, to desired doneness.

3. In a medium mixing bowl, combine romaine with sesame oil and remaining ginger and vinegar; toss to coat.

4. Split dressed lettuce between 2 salad bowls, top with tuna steaks, and garnish with chopped green onions.

PER SERVING | Calories: 386 | Fat: 22 g | Protein: 36 g | Sodium: 578 mg | Fiber: 2 g | Carbohydrates: 10 g | Sugar: 2 g

Salad Niçoise

This is a hearty tuna salad that doesn't contain any artificial or gut-damaging toppings. The tangy dressing will surprise you.

INGREDIENTS | SERVES 2

2 cups Idaho potatoes, peeled

1 cup green beans, trimmed

3 tablespoons extra-virgin olive oil

1 tablespoon white balsamic vinegar

1 teaspoon dry mustard

1 (5-ounce) can solid white albacore tuna in water, drained

4 medium tomatoes, wedged

½ cup sliced black or green olives

2 tablespoons capers, rinsed

Try New Things

Just like children, sometimes adults think they know what they like and what they don't, and they don't deviate from their tastes. However, you may be pleasantly surprised when you try something you thought you wouldn't like. So just like you tell your kids—*try* it and see if you like it!

1. Boil peeled potatoes in a pot of water until fork tender. When cool, cut into cubes.

2. Fill another pot with water and bring to a boil. While pot is heating, prepare an ice bath by filling a bowl with cold water and ice. Place green beans into boiling water and let sit for 2 minutes. Remove green beans from heat and place them into the ice bath immediately. Remove beans from the ice bath as soon as they feel cool to the touch.

3. In a large mixing bowl, whisk together olive oil, vinegar, and mustard.

4. Add tuna, tomato wedges, boiled potatoes, blanched green beans, olives, and capers. Mix well and serve.

PER SERVING | Calories: 485 | Fat: 28 g | Protein: 23 g | Sodium: 608 mg | Fiber: 10 g | Carbohydrates: 40 g | Sugar: 9 g

Romaine and Avocado Salad

A cup of sliced raw green bell pepper contains 12 percent of your daily value (DV) of vitamin A, but an equivalent cup of sliced red bell peppers contains 104 percent DV! Red bell peppers provide both color and taste to your meals, along with plenty of both vitamins C and A.

INGREDIENTS | SERVES 4

Salad

1 large head romaine lettuce
1 large tomato, chopped
1 small red bell pepper, cut into 1" strips
½ small avocado, cut into chunks
2 tablespoons unsweetened dried cranberries

Dressing

2 tablespoons fresh lemon juice
2 teaspoons balsamic vinegar, no sulfites added
1 tablespoon extra-virgin olive oil

For Garnish

2 tablespoons coarsely chopped walnuts or almonds (optional)

1. Remove outer leaves of lettuce head and discard. Chop inner leaves. Rinse in cold water and dry with paper towels.

2. Place lettuce in a large bowl and add remaining salad ingredients.

3. Whisk together dressing ingredients in a small bowl.

4. Toss salad with dressing.

5. Sprinkle with chopped walnuts or almonds, if desired.

PER SERVING | Calories: 121 | Fat: 9 g | Protein: 2 g | Sodium: 457 mg | Fiber: 4 g | Carbohydrates: 11 g | Sugar: 5 g

Spicy Eggs with Romaine and Arugula

Hard-boiled eggs sprinkled with tasty spices provide a protein-rich topping on this crisp salad. These flavors are the perfect answer if your salads have gotten boring!

INGREDIENTS | SERVES 2

2 tablespoons red wine vinegar

1 tablespoon extra-virgin olive oil

1 teaspoon all-natural sea salt

1 teaspoon ground black pepper

1½ cups chopped romaine lettuce

1½ cups chopped arugula

1 teaspoon ground cayenne pepper

4 large hard-boiled eggs, cut in half lengthwise

1. In a medium mixing bowl, whisk together vinegar, olive oil, salt, and pepper until well blended.

2. Add lettuce and arugula to bowl and toss to coat with dressing mixture.

3. Sprinkle cayenne evenly over cut side of eggs.

4. Divide salad between 2 serving bowls and top with egg halves.

PER SERVING | Calories: 221 | Fat: 17 g | Protein: 14 g | Sodium: 1,328 mg | Fiber: 2 g | Carbohydrates: 4 g | Sugar: 2 g

Protein-Packed Salads

If you try to incorporate complex carbs, lean proteins, and healthy fats at every meal, you'll see just how versatile salads can be. By topping crunchy lettuce of any type with eggs, lean chicken, beef, or fish and tossing it with extra-virgin olive oil, you've created a food combination of every important macronutrient your body needs.

Fruit Salad with Ginger and Lemon Juice

Traditional fruit salad is normally just a few fruits and melons thrown together, tossed, and served. These delicious ingredients get tossed in a tasty dressing of freshly squeezed lemon juice and minced ginger for a heightened flavor experience that will transform your fruit salad into something completely new and wonderful.

INGREDIENTS | SERVES 4

1 grapefruit, sectioned

1 cup pineapple chunks

1 cup sliced green seedless grapes

1 Granny Smith apple, cored, sliced, and chopped

1 cup cubed cantaloupe

1 cup cubed honeydew melon

3 tablespoons fresh lemon juice

2 tablespoons minced ginger

In a large mixing bowl, toss together all ingredients to coat and combine thoroughly. Chill in refrigerator and then serve.

PER SERVING | Calories: 127 | Fat: 1 g | Protein: 2 g | Sodium: 18 mg | Fiber: 3 g | Carbohydrates: 32 g | Sugar: 25 g

Grilled Eggplant Salad

This salad is best served cold and is even tastier the next day after the flavors of the eggplant and tomato mixture have a chance to coalesce.

INGREDIENTS | SERVES 4

2 tablespoons plus ½ teaspoon all-natural sea salt, divided

1 large eggplant

2 medium tomatoes, diced

1 small bunch fresh flat-leaf parsley, finely chopped

2 medium cloves garlic, minced

⅛ teaspoon ground black pepper

1 tablespoon dried oregano

¼ cup extra-virgin olive oil, divided

1. Slice eggplant into disks ¼" thick. Fill a large mixing bowl or pot with water, add 2 tablespoons salt, and mix well; place eggplant disks in salt bath and set a heavy plate on top to weigh them down. Let soak for 25 minutes. Mix periodically to ensure salty water soaks into eggplant completely.

2. In a small bowl, combine tomatoes, parsley, garlic, salt, pepper, oregano, and 3 tablespoons olive oil; mix well and set aside.

3. Preheat grill on high. When hot, spray or wipe with vegetable oil.

4. Brush (or spray) one side of each eggplant slice with a little olive oil; place oiled-side down across grill, starting from top left rear section and filling entire surface in rows. Brush (or spray) a little olive oil on top of eggplant slices. Grill until softened, about 6–8 minutes, watching carefully so they don't burn.

5. Brush with olive oil again; turn over. Grill for another 4 minutes; give final brushing of oil. Grill for 1 minute or so.

6. Arrange several eggplant disks on each serving plate, spoon some tomato mixture on top, and sprinkle with oregano.

PER SERVING | Calories: 154 | Fat: 13 g | Protein: 2 g | Sodium: 3,048 mg | Fiber: 5 g | Carbohydrates: 10 g | Sugar: 5 g

Thai Beef Strip Salad

This is a great salad that's packed with marinated steak, fresh ingredients, and delicious aromatic herbs. Unique and definitely different from the usual dinner salad, this makes a great appetizer, side, or main dish.

INGREDIENTS | SERVES 4

2 cups fresh lime juice

½ cup coconut aminos

1 cucumber, peeled and sliced

1 pint cherry tomatoes

½ cup chopped fresh mint

½ cup chopped fresh cilantro

1 cup chopped green onions

1 cup sliced lemongrass (about 1" pieces)

1 pound flank steak

6 cups chopped romaine lettuce

Steak Lovers Rejoice!

If you're a steak lover, you will be happy to hear that lean steak strips atop a beautiful combination of vegetables is one of the best meals you can eat for your gut. Add some homemade dressing and you have a complex carbohydrate, protein, and healthy fat combination that constitutes the perfect meal.

1. Preheat grill on medium and spray with homemade olive oil spray.

2. In a large mixing bowl, combine lime juice, coconut aminos, cucumbers, tomatoes, mint, cilantro, green onions, and lemongrass; mix until well combined.

3. Brush one side of steak with marinade and place seasoned-side down on grill. Cook 7 minutes. Brush unseasoned side with marinade and flip steak. Grill for another 7 minutes or until cooked to desired doneness.

4. Remove steak from grill and let rest for 10 minutes before slicing thinly (about ¼"–½" thick). Place steak slices in marinade, cover, and let soak in refrigerator for at least 1 hour.

5. In a large salad bowl, toss romaine with steak and vegetable combination to coat completely. Serve cold.

PER SERVING | Calories: 235 | Fat: 9 g | Protein: 27 g | Sodium: 2,307 mg | Fiber: 4 g | Carbohydrates: 11 g | Sugar: 5 g

Apple Coleslaw

This coleslaw recipe is a refreshing and sweet alternative to the traditional coleslaw with mayonnaise. The sesame seeds give it a pleasant, nutty flavor.

INGREDIENTS | SERVES 4

2 cups packaged coleslaw mix
1 tart apple, chopped
½ cup chopped celery
½ cup chopped green bell pepper
¼ cup extra-virgin olive oil
2 tablespoons fresh lemon juice
1 tablespoon sesame seeds

1. In a medium bowl, combine coleslaw mix, apple, celery, and bell pepper.

2. In a small bowl, whisk together remaining ingredients. Pour over coleslaw mixture and toss to coat. Chill before serving.

PER SERVING | Calories: 161 | Fat: 14 g | Protein: 1 g | Sodium: 19 mg | Fiber: 3 g | Carbohydrates: 10 g | Sugar: 7 g

Sprinkle on Some Seeds

Sesame seeds may be small, but they pack a nutritional punch. An ounce of sesame seeds contains almost 5 grams of protein and 4 grams of fiber. Sesame seeds are also rich in monounsaturated fatty acids, which can help reduce inflammation and neutralize free radicals.

Endive and Avocado Salad

*The bite from the olives and vinegar are balanced with the refreshing flavors
and textures of fresh tomato and avocado. This amazing salad looks great,
tastes great, and does wonders for your boring lunchtime routine!*

INGREDIENTS | SERVES 2

2 tablespoons extra-virgin olive oil

1 tablespoon red wine vinegar

1 teaspoon all-natural sea salt

1 teaspoon ground black pepper

2 tomatoes, wedged

½ cup sliced black olives

2 cups whole endive leaves

1 avocado, sliced

1. In a large mixing bowl, combine olive oil, vinegar, salt, pepper, tomatoes, and olives; toss well to coat.

2. Divide endive leaves evenly between 2 salad bowls. Top with tomato mixture and garnish with avocado slices.

PER SERVING | Calories: 468 | Fat: 41 g | Protein: 15 g | Sodium: 1,540 mg | Fiber: 10 g | Carbohydrates: 14 g | Sugar: 1 g

Root Vegetable Salad

This root salad has a nice texture and color. It will go well with any traditional fall or winter dish and will make your home smell like a holiday meal.

INGREDIENTS | SERVES 4

1 rutabaga, peeled and cubed

1 turnip, peeled and cubed

6 parsnips, peeled and cubed

3 tablespoons extra-virgin olive oil

1 teaspoon ground cinnamon

3 medium cloves garlic, minced

1 teaspoon ground ginger

1 teaspoon ground black pepper

1. Preheat oven to 400°F.

2. Place rutabaga, turnip, and parsnips in a roasting pan and drizzle with olive oil. Sprinkle with cinnamon, garlic, ginger, and pepper. Toss to coat evenly.

3. Roast for 40–50 minutes, or until fork-tender.

PER SERVING | Calories: 291 | Fat: 11 g | Protein: 4 g | Sodium: 61 mg | Fiber: 13 g | Carbohydrates: 48 g | Sugar: 16 g

Root Vegetables

Roots are underappreciated parts of plants. These underground vegetables are great for gut health, high in vitamin A, and are a nice form of carbohydrate fuel to eat, particularly after exercising.

Tahini Dressing

The flavor of this dressing makes it the perfect addition to any salad, but it goes especially well with salads topped with chicken or turkey.

INGREDIENTS | SERVES 4

2 tablespoons olive oil

2 tablespoons sesame oil

2 tablespoons tahini paste

½ teaspoon ground black pepper

1 teaspoon dried thyme

Combine all ingredients in a small bowl and mix well. Use immediately.

PER SERVING | Calories: 165 | Fat: 18 g | Protein: 1 g | Sodium: 9 mg | Fiber: 1 g | Carbohydrates: 2 g | Sugar: 0 g

Curry Salad Dressing

This dressing has a hint of warm spice from the curry powder that goes well on any salad.

INGREDIENTS | SERVES 4

3 tablespoons olive oil

Juice of 1 medium lime

1 teaspoon curry powder

½ teaspoon ground black pepper

1 teaspoon dried basil

Combine all ingredients in a small bowl and stir well. Serve immediately on salad.

PER SERVING | Calories: 95 | Fat: 11 g | Protein: 0 g | Sodium: 1 mg | Fiber: 0 g | Carbohydrates: 1 g | Sugar: 0 g

Lemon-Dill Dressing

This traditional dressing shouldn't be limited to salads alone; it's great served with your best fish recipes, or double the recipe to make a marinade for grilled chicken.

INGREDIENTS | SERVES 2

2 tablespoons extra-virgin olive oil
Juice of 1 medium lemon
1 teaspoon minced fresh dill
½ teaspoon ground black pepper

Combine all ingredients and mix well. Use immediately.

PER SERVING | Calories: 120 | Fat: 14 g | Protein: 0 g | Sodium: 0 mg | Fiber: 0 g | Carbohydrates: 0 g | Sugar: 0 g

CHAPTER 14

Soups, Stocks, and Sauces

Butternut Squash Chowder

This hearty, savory butternut chowder makes a great meal on its own,
but in smaller portions it also serves as a delicious starter.

INGREDIENTS | SERVES 6

1 medium butternut squash

1 tablespoon melted ghee

4 bacon slices, cut into ½" pieces

1 medium yellow onion, chopped

2 medium stalks celery, chopped

1 dried bay leaf

1 teaspoon chopped fresh sage

4 teaspoons all-natural sea salt

1 teaspoon ground black pepper

2 medium russet potatoes, peeled and cubed

3 cups Basic Chicken Stock (see recipe in this chapter)

½ cup coconut cream

1. Preheat oven to 375°F.

2. Cut squash lengthwise; remove and discard seeds. Place on a large baking sheet, flesh-side up, and brush with melted ghee. Bake for 45 minutes, or until squash is fork-tender. Remove from oven and let cool.

3. In a large skillet, cook bacon over medium heat until crispy. Transfer bacon to paper towels to drain. Crumble bacon and set aside.

4. Pour off all but about 1 tablespoon of bacon fat from skillet. Return skillet to medium heat and add onion, celery, bay leaf, sage, salt, and pepper; sauté for 5 minutes, or until onion is translucent.

5. Add potatoes; cover and cook for 5 minutes, stirring occasionally.

6. Add stock; simmer for 2 minutes, stirring to scrape up browned bits from bottom of pan. Bring to a boil, then reduce heat to low and simmer for 10–15 minutes, or until potatoes are soft.

7. Scoop squash out of skins and purée in a food processor until smooth. Add to stock mixture along with crumbled bacon; simmer for 5 minutes.

8. Stir in coconut cream. Remove and discard bay leaf. Serve hot.

PER SERVING | Calories: 209 | Fat: 10 g | Protein: 4 g | Sodium: 2,033 mg | Fiber: 4 g | Carbohydrates: 22 g | Sugar: 4 g

Creamy Asparagus Soup

Creamy soups are often laden with flour and other ingredients that are not so good for your gut. This version is just as tasty and has the same consistency, but all the ingredients are gut approved!

INGREDIENTS | SERVES 4

2 tablespoons olive oil, divided

1 medium clove garlic, minced

2 small Idaho potatoes, peeled and chopped

2 tablespoons filtered water

2 pounds asparagus, chopped

3 medium leeks, chopped

2 teaspoons ground black pepper

2 cups Homemade Almond Milk (see recipe in Chapter 10)

1. Heat 1 tablespoon olive oil in a stockpot over medium heat. Add garlic and potatoes; sauté for about 10–15 minutes, until potatoes are fork-tender, adding water as needed to prevent sticking and promote steaming.

2. Add remaining olive oil to pan. Add asparagus, leeks, and pepper to stockpot and sauté until tender.

3. Add almond milk to the pot and bring to a boil. Reduce heat to low and simmer for 15 minutes.

4. With an immersion blender, emulsify the ingredients until thick and creamy. Serve immediately.

PER SERVING | Calories: 213 | Fat: 4 g | Protein: 8 g | Sodium: 115 mg | Fiber: 9 g | Carbohydrates: 36 g | Sugar: 8 g

Cranberry-Pear Sauce

This tastes great spooned over oatmeal or on top of a grilled piece of pork.

INGREDIENTS | SERVES 2

2 cups fresh or unsweetened frozen cranberries

1 Gala apple, finely chopped

2 ripe Bartlett pears, finely chopped

1 teaspoon orange zest

1 teaspoon ground cinnamon

1 cup unsweetened orange juice concentrate

Combine all ingredients in a medium saucepan and bring to a simmer over medium heat. Cook about 10 minutes, uncovered, until cranberry skins pop and mixture starts to thicken. Serve immediately.

PER SERVING | Calories: 272 | Fat: 0 g | Protein: 2 g | Sodium: 7 mg | Fiber: 14 g | Carbohydrates: 71 g | Sugar: 44 g

Butternut Curry Soup

This is a delicious soup to serve with a crisp salad. Homemade Almond Milk (see recipe in Chapter 10) or young coconut water are good substitutes for the plain filtered water.

INGREDIENTS | SERVES 2

1 cup peeled and chopped cucumber

2 cups peeled and chopped butternut squash

½ cup chopped red bell pepper

1 cup toasted pine nuts

¼ cup diced leeks

2 teaspoons minced gingerroot

1½ teaspoons curry powder

¼ teaspoon all-natural sea salt

¼ teaspoon ground cayenne pepper

1. In a food processor or blender, process cucumber until liquefied.

2. Gradually add remaining ingredients to blender or food processor and blend until smooth. Add a small amount of filtered water gradually if needed to reach desired consistency.

3. Warm soup in a small saucepan over low heat until steaming, about 15 minutes.

PER SERVING | Calories: 567 | Fat: 48 g | Protein: 12 g | Sodium: 305 mg | Fiber: 8 g | Carbohydrates: 35 g | Sugar: 8 g

Gazpacho

It's best to make gazpacho the day before you plan to serve it so that the flavors will penetrate all the vegetables. It should be served chilled.

INGREDIENTS | SERVES 6

1 (28-ounce) can no-salt-added chopped tomatoes

1 medium green bell pepper, chopped

3 medium tomatoes, peeled and chopped

1 cucumber, peeled and chopped

1 small white onion, chopped

2 tablespoons olive oil

½ teaspoon ground black pepper

½ teaspoon ground paprika

¼ teaspoon ground cayenne pepper

1 teaspoon chopped fresh chives

2 teaspoons chopped fresh flat-leaf parsley

½ medium clove garlic, minced

1½ tablespoons fresh lemon juice

1. Blend canned tomatoes in blender until smooth. Pour into a large bowl.

2. Add remaining ingredients to bowl and mix together.

3. Refrigerate at least 12 hours, then serve.

PER SERVING | Calories: 101 | Fat: 5 g | Protein: 3 g | Sodium: 14 mg | Fiber: 4 g | Carbohydrates: 13 g | Sugar: 8 g

Basic Vegetable Stock

Try adding mushrooms, parsnips, garlic, or bell peppers for additional flavor in this hearty stock.

INGREDIENTS | MAKES 1 GALLON (½-CUP SERVINGS)

2 pounds yellow onions
1 pound carrots
1 pound celery
1 small bunch fresh parsley
1½ gallons filtered water
4 sprigs fresh thyme
2 dried bay leaves
15 peppercorns

Homemade Stocks

Your homemade stocks add a special quality to all the dishes you add them to. Not only is the flavor of homemade stocks better than that from purchased bases, but they don't contain any artificial ingredients or preservatives. Always cook stocks uncovered, as covering them will cause the liquid to become cloudy.

1. Peel and roughly chop onions and carrots. Roughly chop celery (stalks only; no leaves) and parsley stems.

2. Add vegetables and water to a large stockpot over medium heat; bring to a simmer and cook, uncovered, for 1½ hours.

3. Add herbs and peppercorns; simmer, uncovered, for 45 minutes. Adjust seasonings to taste as necessary.

4. Remove from heat and cool by submerging the pot in an ice-water bath. Place in freezer-safe containers and store in freezer until ready to use.

PER SERVING | Calories: 15 | Fat: 0 g | Protein: 0 g | Sodium: 0 mg | Fiber: 0 g | Carbohydrates: 3 g | Sugar: 2 g

Basic Chicken Stock

You can use fresh bay leaves instead of dry in this recipe, but remember to double the quantity to get the same concentrated flavor of dry herbs.

INGREDIENTS | MAKES 1 GALLON (½-CUP SERVINGS)

2 pounds yellow onions
1 pound carrots
1 pound celery
1 small bunch fresh flat-leaf parsley
4 pounds skinless, bone-in chicken
1½ gallons filtered water
4 sprigs fresh thyme
2 dried bay leaves
15 peppercorns

1. Peel and chop onions and carrots. Chop celery (stalks only; no leaves) and parsley.

2. Add chicken, vegetables, and water to a large stockpot over medium heat; bring to simmer and cook, uncovered, for 5 hours.

3. Add herbs and peppercorns; simmer, uncovered, for 45 minutes.

4. Remove from heat. Strain and discard solids. Cool by submerging the pot in an ice-water bath. Remove all chicken fat that solidifies at the surface before using or freezing. Place in freezer-safe containers and store in freezer until ready to use.

PER SERVING | Calories: 19 | Fat: 1 g | Protein: 3 g | Sodium: 0 mg | Fiber: 0 g | Carbohydrates: 4 g | Sugar: 2 g

Beef Stock

Always thoroughly cool the stock and remove solidified fat from the top before using or freezing.

INGREDIENTS | MAKES 1 GALLON (½-CUP SERVINGS)

3 large yellow onions
½ pound carrots
3 large stalks celery
1 small bunch fresh flat-leaf parsley
1 tablespoon olive oil
5 pounds bone-in beef shank
1½ gallons filtered water
4 sprigs fresh thyme
2 dried bay leaves
15 peppercorns

The Fond

The residue left in the bottom of the pan when making stock is known as fond. If you find you cannot release it all, return the pan to the stovetop, add a small amount of water, and whisk to remove; then add it to the stock. The fond has a high concentration of flavor and should not be discarded.

1. Preheat oven to 400°F.

2. Peel and roughly chop onions and carrots. Chop celery (stalks only; no leaves) and parsley.

3. Place oil, beef, and vegetables in a large roasting pan; bake for 30–45 minutes, until well browned.

4. Transfer meat and vegetables to a large stockpot with water. Gently scrape the bottom of the roasting pan to loosen all residue and add it to the stockpot. Simmer over medium heat, uncovered, for 8–10 hours.

5. Add herbs and peppercorns; simmer, uncovered, for 30 minutes.

6. Remove from heat. Strain and discard solids. Cool by submerging the pot in an ice-water bath. Place in freezer-safe containers and store in the freezer until ready to use.

PER SERVING | Calories: 19 | Fat: 0 g | Protein: 1 g | Sodium: 0 mg | Fiber: 0 g | Carbohydrates: 4 g | Sugar: 3 g

Seafood Stock

Seafood shells, such as those from lobster and shrimp, are ideal for making a seafood stock. Be sure to thoroughly clean the leek before adding it to the stockpot.

INGREDIENTS | MAKES 1 GALLON (½-CUP SERVINGS)

4 pounds seafood shells

3 large yellow onions

¼ pound shallots

1 large leek

½ pound parsnips

2 medium stalks celery

1 small bunch fresh flat-leaf parsley

1 cup Basic Vegetable Stock (see recipe in this chapter)

1½ gallons filtered water

4 springs fresh thyme

2 dried bay leaves

15 peppercorns

Make It Juicy

Instead of vegetable stock, you could substitute unsweetened apple juice or grape juice for a sweeter flavor in this recipe. Different vegetables, like bell peppers and carrots, can sweeten this stock as well.

1. Thoroughly rinse seafood shells in ice-cold water. Peel and roughly chop onions, shallots, leek, and parsnips. Chop celery (stalks only; no leaves) and parsley.

2. Place shells, vegetables, stock, and water in a large stockpot over medium heat; bring to a simmer and cook, uncovered, for 2 hours.

3. Add herbs and peppercorns; simmer, uncovered, for 30 minutes.

4. Remove from heat. Strain and discard solids. Cool by submerging the pot in an ice-water bath. Place in freezer-safe containers and store in freezer until ready to use.

PER SERVING | Calories: 15 | Fat: 0 g | Protein: 0 g | Sodium: 0 mg | Fiber: 0 g | Carbohydrates: 4 g | Sugar: 2 g

Bone Broth

The gelatin in bone broth helps heal the lining of the digestive tract, which contributes to reversing leaky gut. The key to getting a gelatinous bone broth is allowing your bone broth to cook on low for 24 hours.

INGREDIENTS | MAKES 1 GALLON (½-CUP SERVINGS)

1 large yellow onion
3 medium carrots
3 medium celery stalks
6 garlic cloves
4 pounds beef or pork marrow bones
2 tablespoons apple cider vinegar
3 dried bay leaves
15 peppercorns

1. Coarsely chop onion, carrots, celery, and garlic cloves and add them to the bottom of a 6-quart slow cooker.

2. Place marrow bones on top of the chopped vegetables and pour apple cider vinegar over the bones. Fill slow cooker with just enough water to cover bones.

3. Add bay leaves and peppercorns.

4. Cover slow cooker and set it to low. Let simmer in the slow cooker for 24 hours.

5. Strain and discard solids. Cool by submerging the pot in an ice-water bath. Place in freezer-safe containers and store in freezer until ready to use.

PER SERVING | Calories: 19 | Fat: 0 g | Protein: 1 g | Sodium: 0 mg | Fiber: 0 g | Carbohydrates: 4 g | Sugar: 3 g

Spaghetti Sauce

A combination of fresh and canned tomatoes creates a real depth of flavor in this simple recipe. It freezes very well.

INGREDIENTS | MAKES 1½ QUARTS (½-CUP SERVINGS)

2 tablespoons olive oil

1 medium yellow onion, chopped

3 medium cloves garlic, minced

1 cup chopped button or cremini mushrooms

1 cup peeled and shredded carrots

1 (28-ounce) can diced tomatoes, undrained

1 (6-ounce) can tomato paste

6 plum tomatoes, chopped

1½ cups filtered water

1 teaspoon dried basil

½ teaspoon dried oregano

½ teaspoon all-natural sea salt

¼ teaspoon ground black pepper

1 dried bay leaf

1. Heat olive oil in a large, heavy saucepan; cook onion and garlic over medium heat until tender, 5–6 minutes. Add mushrooms and carrots; cook 4–5 minutes longer.

2. Add remaining ingredients to saucepan. Bring to a boil, then reduce heat to low. Cover and simmer for 45–50 minutes, until sauce is blended and slightly thickened. Remove bay leaf and discard.

3. Serve immediately or cover and refrigerate up to 4 days. Freeze for longer storage.

PER SERVING | Calories: 68 | Fat: 3 g | Protein: 2 g | Sodium: 129 mg | Fiber: 3 g | Carbohydrates: 12 g | Sugar: 7 g

Tomatillo Salsa

Salsa verde (green salsa) is usually made with roasted bell peppers.
This version, made with tomatillos, is tangy and spicy.

INGREDIENTS | MAKES 2 CUPS (¼-CUP SERVINGS)

¾ pound tomatillos, husked
1 medium jalapeño pepper
1 medium habanero pepper
½ cup filtered water
1 tablespoon olive oil
4 medium cloves garlic, minced
1 large white onion, chopped
½ teaspoon all-natural sea salt
¼ teaspoon ground black pepper
½ cup chopped fresh cilantro
¼ cup chopped fresh flat-leaf parsley

Tomatillos

Tomatillos are small green fruit with a papery covering. Remove the covering and rinse before using. They are not green tomatoes; in fact, they are a type of berry, related to the gooseberry. They can be eaten raw or cooked, although cooking does make them a bit less tart and crunchy.

1. Rinse tomatillos and coarsely chop. Combine in a medium saucepan with jalapeño and habanero peppers and water; bring to a boil. Reduce heat and simmer, stirring frequently, for 5 minutes. Remove from heat, drain, and set aside.

2. In medium skillet, heat olive oil over medium heat. Add garlic and onion; cook until onion is crisp-tender, about 5–6 minutes, stirring frequently. Remove from heat.

3. In a blender or food processor, combine tomatillo mixture and remaining ingredients. Blend or process to desired consistency. Cover and chill in refrigerator for at least 2 hours to blend flavors. Will last for 2–3 days, covered, in fridge.

PER SERVING | Calories: 41 | Fat: 2 g | Protein: 1 g | Sodium: 148 mg | Fiber: 1 g | Carbohydrates: 5 g | Sugar: 1 g

Walnut-Parsley Pesto

Walnuts add a significant blast of omega-3 fatty acids to this delicious pesto. Toss with spiralized zucchini "noodles" or put a spoonful on top of your eggs in the morning.

INGREDIENTS | SERVES 4

½ cup walnuts

8 medium cloves garlic

1 large bunch fresh flat-leaf parsley, roughly chopped

¼ cup extra-virgin olive oil

⅛ teaspoon ground black pepper

Pesto for All

Pesto is a generic term for anything made by pounding. Most people are familiar with traditional pesto, which is made with basil and pine nuts, but many prefer this variation with parsley and walnuts.

1. Chop walnuts in a food processor or blender. Add garlic and process to form a paste. Add parsley and pulse into walnut mixture.

2. While the blender is running, drizzle in oil until the mixture is smooth. Add pepper, adjusting seasoning to taste. Store in fridge for up to 4 days.

PER SERVING | Calories: 229 | Fat: 23 g | Protein: 3 g | Sodium: 6 mg | Fiber: 1 g | Carbohydrates: 4 g | Sugar: 0 g

Ladolemono (Olive Oil and Lemon Sauce)

This is a classic Greek sauce used on grilled meats, vegetables, and fish.

**INGREDIENTS | MAKES 1 CUP
(1-TABLESPOON
SERVINGS)**

½ cup extra-virgin olive oil

½ cup fresh lemon juice

1 tablespoon dried oregano

1 teaspoon all-natural sea salt

1 teaspoon ground black pepper

In a small bowl, combine all ingredients and mix well. Serve immediately.

PER SERVING | Calories: 61 | Fat: 7 g | Protein: 0 g |
Sodium: 146 mg | Fiber: 0 g | Carbohydrates: 0 g | Sugar: 0 g

Antioxidants for Everyone

Lemon juice, which is an ingredient in almost every Greek dish, is not only a good source of vitamin C, but it also packs a respectable dose of antioxidants. Drizzle it liberally!

Simple Chicken Soup

Soups are a great opportunity to clean out the refrigerator of vegetables and also a good way to add a wider variety of vegetables to your family's diet. Try diced red potato, celery, carrots, parsnips, or mushrooms.

INGREDIENTS | SERVES 4

2 cups each of 2 vegetables of your choice, such as carrots, celery, zucchini, or onions

4 cups Basic Chicken Stock (see recipe in this chapter)

2 cups shredded roast chicken

1 teaspoon minced garlic

¼ cup diced yellow onion

1 tablespoon dried Italian seasoning

1. In a large stockpot, boil vegetables in stock until tender.

2. Add chicken, garlic, onion, and Italian seasoning.

3. Simmer for 30 minutes and serve.

PER SERVING | Calories: 224 | Fat: 11 g | Protein: 21 g | Sodium: 866 mg | Fiber: 2 g | Carbohydrates: 9 g | Sugar: 5 g

Carrot-Thyme Soup

If your carrots are not sweet enough for your taste, try adding a sweet potato to this easy recipe.

INGREDIENTS | SERVES 6

2 pounds carrots

1 large Vidalia onion

4 medium Yukon gold potatoes

3 medium cloves garlic

4 sprigs fresh thyme

1 tablespoon olive oil

6 cups Basic Vegetable Stock (see recipe in this chapter)

½ teaspoon sea salt

⅛ teaspoon ground black pepper

Sweating Vegetables

The term *to sweat* refers to the cooking process by which the product is cooked slowly until softened but not browned.

1. Peel and dice carrots, onion, and potatoes. Mince garlic. Remove thyme leaves from stems; discard stems.

2. Place carrots, onions, potatoes, and garlic in a large stockpot with olive oil. Sweat slowly on medium-low for about 10 minutes, until vegetables are softened.

3. Increase heat to medium, add stock and bring to a simmer; cook, uncovered, for 1 hour.

4. Let mixture cool slightly, then purée in a blender until smooth. Return purée to stockpot and add thyme, salt, and pepper; cook, uncovered, over low heat for another 30 minutes. Serve warm.

PER SERVING | Calories: 200 | Fat: 3 g | Protein: 5 g | Sodium: 391 mg | Fiber: 8 g | Carbohydrates: 41 g | Sugar: 11 g

Rich Broccoli Soup

You don't have to avoid creamy soup if you can't have dairy. Blending makes this soup rich and creamy.

INGREDIENTS | SERVES 4

1 (16-ounce) bag frozen chopped broccoli

3 medium red potatoes, peeled and chopped

1 small Vidalia onion, diced

1 teaspoon fresh lemon juice

1 teaspoon dried Italian seasoning

½ teaspoon all-natural sea salt

⅛ teaspoon ground black pepper

3 cups Basic Vegetable Stock (see recipe in this chapter)

1 cup coconut milk

1. In a medium saucepan on medium-high, combine broccoli, potatoes, onion, lemon juice, seasonings, and stock.

2. Bring to a boil, then reduce heat and simmer, uncovered, for 30 minutes or until potatoes are tender. Let cool slightly before blending.

3. In a blender, combine contents of saucepan with coconut milk. (Or, use an immersion blender to blend in the saucepan.) Blend until smooth, then serve.

PER SERVING | Calories: 311 | Fat: 15 g | Protein: 9 g | Sodium: 145 mg | Fiber: 8 g | Carbohydrates: 40 g | Sugar: 8 g

Carrot-Parsnip Bisque

This Carrot-Parsnip Bisque can be served hot or cold. It's great as an appetizer when entertaining, or for lunch with a crisp green salad on the side.

INGREDIENTS | SERVES 6

6 medium carrots, peeled and sliced

4 medium parsnips, peeled and sliced

1 tablespoon coconut oil

½ cup minced shallots

½ teaspoon ground white pepper

1 teaspoon all-natural sea salt

1 teaspoon arrowroot or tapioca powder

1 cup Basic Vegetable Stock (see recipe in this chapter)

2 cups coconut milk

½ cup finely chopped fresh basil

½ teaspoon ground nutmeg

1. In a steamer over medium heat, cook carrots and parsnips until soft, about 10 minutes.

2. In a large stockpot, heat coconut oil; add shallots, pepper, and salt. Sauté for 5 minutes, or until shallots are tender. Sprinkle in arrowroot or tapioca powder and whisk in stock; stir constantly until mixture thickens and comes to a boil, about 3 minutes.

3. In a food processor or blender, combine stock mixture with steamed carrots and parsnips; purée until smooth.

4. Add coconut milk; process until well mixed, and return to pot.

5. Stir in basil and nutmeg; heat on low, stirring occasionally for 1 minute, or until heated through. Serve hot, or chill in refrigerator and serve cold.

PER SERVING | Calories: 225 | Fat: 19 g | Protein: 3 g | Sodium: 626 mg | Fiber: 3 g | Carbohydrates: 15 g | Sugar: 10 g

Butternut Squash Soup

This soup is a scrumptious treat on a cool fall day. Warm family and friends with a delightful blend of aroma and flavor.

INGREDIENTS | SERVES 4

1 pound butternut squash

1 tablespoon olive oil

1 medium Vidalia onion, chopped

½ cup flax meal

4 cups Basic Chicken Stock (see recipe in this chapter)

1 cup Homemade Almond Milk (see recipe in Chapter 10)

½ teaspoon ground cinnamon

¼ teaspoon ground cloves

¼ teaspoon ground nutmeg

1. Peel and seed squash, then chop into 1" cubes.

2. In a large stockpot or Dutch oven, heat olive oil over medium-high heat. Sauté onion and squash for 5 minutes.

3. Add flax meal and stock, and increase heat to high. Bring to boil, then reduce heat to low and simmer for 45 minutes.

4. In batches, purée squash mixture in blender or food processor and return to pot.

5. Stir in almond milk, cinnamon, cloves, and nutmeg. Serve hot.

PER SERVING | Calories: 182 | Fat: 9 g | Protein: 9 g | Sodium: 495 mg | Fiber: 6 g | Carbohydrates: 20 g | Sugar: 6 g

Roasted Root Vegetable Soup

This recipe works well a hearty side dish or as an entrée. To vary the flavors in this dish, try substituting the parsnips with turnips and the potatoes with sweet potatoes or butternut squash.

INGREDIENTS | SERVES 6

2 medium parsnips

3 medium carrots

2 large Yukon gold potatoes

3 medium stalks celery

3 medium yellow onions

1 tablespoon olive oil

1 sprig fresh rosemary

4 cups Basic Vegetable Stock (see recipe in this chapter)

3 sprigs fresh thyme

¼ small bunch fresh flat-leaf parsley

2 dried bay leaves

⅛ teaspoon ground black pepper

All-natural sea salt to taste (optional)

1. Preheat oven to 375°F.

2. Peel (as necessary) and chop all vegetables.

3. Pour oil into a large roasting pan. Place vegetables and rosemary sprig in pan and roast until al dente, about 30–45 minutes. Remove from oven, discard rosemary sprig, and let cool slightly.

4. In a blender, purée roasted vegetables thoroughly in small batches, adding stock to each batch and processing until smooth. Pour purée into a large stockpot and bring to a simmer over medium heat.

5. Chop thyme leaves (discard stems) and parsley. Add to stockpot along with remaining ingredients; simmer for 45 minutes. Serve.

PER SERVING (without sea salt) | Calories: 151 | Fat: 3 g | Protein: 3 g | Sodium: 118 mg | Fiber: 7 g | Carbohydrates: 30 g | Sugar: 8 g

Cream of Cauliflower Soup

Cauliflower is a fantastic vegetable because of its versatility. Blended cauliflower can be used as a thickener in recipes that call for potatoes or root vegetables.

INGREDIENTS | SERVES 4

1 large head cauliflower, chopped

3 medium stalks celery, chopped

1 medium carrot, peeled and chopped

2 medium cloves garlic, minced

1 large Vidalia onion, chopped

2 teaspoons ground cumin

½ teaspoon ground black pepper

1 tablespoon chopped fresh flat-leaf parsley

¼ teaspoon dried dill weed

1. In a large stockpot or Dutch oven, combine cauliflower, celery, carrot, garlic, onion, cumin, and pepper.

2. Add water to just cover ingredients in pot. Bring to a boil over high heat.

3. Reduce heat to low. Simmer about 8 minutes or until vegetables are tender.

4. Stir in parsley and dill before serving.

PER SERVING | Calories: 90 | Fat: 1 g | Protein: 6 g | Sodium: 114 mg | Fiber: 7 g | Carbohydrates: 20 g | Sugar: 8 g

Curried Zucchini Soup

Five cups of chopped zucchini equals about 6 baby zucchini, 2–3 medium-sized ones, or 1 jumbo backyard garden variety.

INGREDIENTS | SERVES 8

1 tablespoon olive oil

5 cups chopped zucchini

2 medium yellow onions, chopped

1 medium stalk celery, diced

1 medium clove garlic, minced

2 teaspoons curry powder

¾ teaspoon all-natural sea salt

½ teaspoon ground cinnamon

¼ teaspoon ground black pepper

6 cups Basic Vegetable Stock (see recipe in this chapter)

1. In a large stockpot, heat olive oil over medium heat; sauté zucchini, onions, celery, and garlic with curry powder, salt, cinnamon, and pepper, stirring occasionally, for about 10 minutes, until vegetables are softened.

2. Pour in stock. Bring to a boil, then reduce to a simmer. Cook, covered, for 20 minutes, or until vegetables are very tender.

3. In a blender or food processor, purée soup in batches until smooth. Pour into a clean stockpot and reheat, but do not boil. Season with more salt and pepper to taste if desired.

PER SERVING | Calories: 72 | Fat: 3 g | Protein: 5 g | Sodium: 285 mg | Fiber: 2 g | Carbohydrates: 8 g | Sugar: 4 g

Pumpkin Soup

This is a perfect autumn soup to celebrate the harvest season. If you're short on time or pumpkins are out of season, substitute 1 (15-ounce) can of puréed pumpkin for the fresh pumpkin.

INGREDIENTS | SERVES 6

2 cups flesh from a sugar pumpkin, diced, seeds reserved

1 teaspoon all-natural sea salt

3 medium leeks, sliced

1½ teaspoons minced gingerroot

1 tablespoon olive oil

½ teaspoon lemon zest

1 teaspoon fresh lemon juice

2 quarts Basic Vegetable Stock (see recipe in this chapter)

⅛ teaspoon ground black pepper

1 tablespoon extra-virgin olive oil, for drizzling

Zesting

If you don't have a zester, you can still easily make lemon zest. Simply use your cheese grater, but be careful to grate only the rind and not the white pith, which tends to be bitter.

1. Preheat oven to 375°F.

2. Clean pumpkin seeds thoroughly by rinsing them under running water and removing any pulp. Place seeds on a baking sheet and sprinkle with salt. Roast for 5–8 minutes, until light golden. Set aside.

3. Spread cubed pumpkin in a 9" × 13" baking dish with leeks, ginger, and olive oil, and toss to coat; roast for 45–60 minutes, until cooked al dente.

4. Transfer cooked pumpkin mixture to a large stockpot and add zest, juice, stock, and pepper; let simmer for 45 minutes.

5. To serve, ladle into serving bowls. Drizzle with extra-virgin olive oil and sprinkle with toasted pumpkin seeds.

PER SERVING | Calories: 100 | Fat: 4 g | Protein: 3 g | Sodium: 62 mg | Fiber: 2 g | Carbohydrates: 10 g | Sugar: 7 g

CHAPTER 15

Snacks

Great Guacamole

Full of flavor and healthy fats, this chunky dip is satisfying and nutritious. Beautiful colors from all the fresh ingredients make this delectable delight a feast for your eyes and your taste buds.

INGREDIENTS | SERVES 12

3 large ripe avocados, mashed to desired consistency

½ medium red onion, chopped

2 large Roma tomatoes, chopped

2 tablespoons chopped fresh cilantro

1 medium clove garlic, crushed

¼ cup fresh lime juice

1 teaspoon all-natural sea salt

1 teaspoon ground black pepper

Combine all ingredients in a small mixing bowl and blend thoroughly. Serve immediately.

PER SERVING | Calories: 84 | Fat: 7 g | Protein: 1.2 g | Sodium: 200 mg | Fiber: 4 g | Carbohydrates: 5 g | Sugar: 1 g

Avocados: Nature's Best Form of Healthy Fat

This fruit, a member of the pear family, is not only rich in vitamins and minerals, it's also packed with healthy fats that multitask for your body. Brimming with vitamins A, C, and E, avocados are great for improving the performance of the brain, digestive system, and metabolism.

Papaya Salsa

Look for a papaya that is firm and has a nice yellow color, not green. Cut a ripe papaya in half, scoop out the seeds, and cut into bite-sized pieces.

INGREDIENTS | SERVES 4

1 cup diced mango

1 large banana, sliced

1 cup diced papaya

3 tablespoons fresh lime juice

1 tablespoon extra-virgin olive oil

1 teaspoon all-natural sea salt

1 tablespoon chopped fresh mint

Toss together fruit, lime juice, and olive oil in a medium bowl. Season with salt, and stir to combine. Sprinkle with chopped mint leaves before serving.

PER SERVING | Calories: 117 | Fat: 4 g | Protein: 1 g | Sodium: 586 mg | Fiber: 3 g | Carbohydrates: 22 g | Sugar: 15 g

Spiced Cinnamon-Cranberry Applesauce

This is a flavorful twist on traditional applesauce. This dish is great served as a snack, or as a sauce on your favorite roast pork, chicken, or turkey recipes.

INGREDIENTS | SERVES 4

8 Gala apples

1 cup fresh or unsweetened frozen cranberries

2 teaspoons ground cinnamon

½ teaspoon ground cloves

⅛ teaspoon ground nutmeg

Cranberry Warning

Large quantities of either cranberry juice or cranberry capsules may cause diarrhea in people with irritable bowel syndrome (IBS), so limit your intake if you experience symptoms of IBS.

1. Peel, core, and chop apples.

2. Place cranberries and apples in 4-quart slow cooker. Stir in cinnamon and cloves.

3. Cover and cook on low for 4 hours or until cranberries and apples are very soft.

4. Add nutmeg and stir to mix.

PER SERVING | Calories: 204 | Fat: 0 g | Protein: 0 g | Sodium: 5 mg | Fiber: 11 g | Carbohydrates: 54 g | Sugar: 39 g

Deviled Eggs

This is a quick recipe that you can whip up in no time. Both kids and adults will love these, and they can be easily served at parties or family gatherings.

INGREDIENTS | SERVES 10

10 large hard-boiled eggs
2 medium green onions, finely chopped
2 medium cloves garlic, minced
1 medium stalk celery, finely chopped
1 teaspoon dry mustard
1 teaspoon ground black pepper
½ teaspoon ground sweet paprika

1. Peel eggs, cut in half lengthwise, and separate yolks from whites.

2. Combine egg yolks, onions, garlic, celery, dry mustard, and pepper. Mix well to form a paste.

3. Stuff egg whites with yolk mixture.

4. Sprinkle paprika over eggs and serve.

PER SERVING | Calories: 76 | Fat: 5 g | Protein: 7 g | Sodium: 63 mg | Fiber: 0 g | Carbohydrates: 2 g | Sugar: 0 g

Baked Apples

You will feel as if you're eating apple pie when you eat these, and your house will smell like Thanksgiving dinner whenever you make them.

INGREDIENTS | SERVES 6

6 Pink Lady apples
1 cup unsweetened coconut flakes
⅛ teaspoon ground cinnamon

1. Preheat oven to 350°F.

2. Hollow out apples by removing top portion of cores, leaving apples intact with ½" of core at bottom.

3. Place apples in a medium baking dish. Fill hollows with coconut flakes and sprinkle with cinnamon.

4. Bake for 10–15 minutes, until apples are completely soft and lightly browned on top.

PER SERVING | Calories: 215 | Fat: 11 g | Protein: 1 g | Sodium: 8 mg | Fiber: 7 g | Carbohydrates: 29 g | Sugar: 20 g

Cinnamon Toasted Butternut Squash

This side dish or snack is a great fall dish. It smells amazing and will give you the carbohydrate boost your body needs.

INGREDIENTS | SERVES 4

3 cups cubed butternut squash
1 teaspoon ground cinnamon
1 teaspoon ground nutmeg

1. Preheat oven to 350°F.

2. Place squash in a 9" × 11" baking dish. Sprinkle with cinnamon and nutmeg.

3. Bake for 30 minutes or until tender and lightly browned.

PER SERVING │ Calories: 48 │ Fat: 0 g │ Protein: 1 g │ Sodium: 4 mg │ Fiber: 2 g │ Carbohydrates: 13 g │ Sugar: 3 g

Sardines in Red Pepper Boats

These boats can be put together in a few minutes and are ideal snacks for transporting. Additionally, this dish is a great source of omega-3s.

INGREDIENTS | SERVES 2

1 (3.75-ounce) can no-salt-added, skinless, boneless sardines

1 medium red bell pepper

Juice of 1 medium lemon

⅛ teaspoon ground black pepper

1. Drain sardines.

2. Cut the stemmed top off the bell pepper and cut bell pepper in half lengthwise; remove ribs and seeds; fill with sardines.

3. Sprinkle with lemon juice and pepper. Serve immediately.

PER SERVING | Calories: 86 | Fat: 4 g | Protein: 9 g | Sodium: 104 mg | Fiber: 1 g | Carbohydrates: 4 g | Sugar: 3 g

Nutty Chocolate Trail Mix

*When you're craving something sweet, throw this quick trail mix
together for a healthy alternative to a chocolate bar.*

INGREDIENTS | SERVES 4

8 ounces organic turkey jerky
½ cup macadamia nuts
½ cup walnuts
½ cup unsweetened coconut flakes
½ cup cacao nibs

1. Cut up turkey jerky into bite-sized pieces and place in a medium bowl.

2. Add remaining ingredients to bowl, mix, and serve. Store in airtight container for up to 2 weeks.

PER SERVING | Calories: 549 | Fat: 34 g | Protein: 23 g | Sodium: 1,058 mg | Fiber: 5 g | Carbohydrates: 20 g | Sugar: 2 g

Blueberry Trail Mix

This trail mix recipe is the perfect blend of fruit and nuts to quiet any hunger pangs. The antioxidants help fight free radicals, while the fatty acids in the seeds provide an anti-inflammatory effect.

INGREDIENTS | SERVES 2

¼ cup unsweetened dried blueberries

¼ cup pumpkin seeds

1 ounce unsalted almonds

⅛ teaspoon ground cinnamon

Combine all ingredients in a 1-quart resealable plastic bag, shake, and enjoy.

PER SERVING | Calories: 241 | Fat: 19 g | Protein: 13 g | Sodium: 6 mg | Fiber: 3 g | Carbohydrates: 23 g | Sugar: 9 g

Antioxidants

Antioxidants are important for attacking free radicals in your body. You really can't eat enough foods containing these important compounds. Feel free to mix up the type of berry you add to this mix. Dehydrated varieties are often available in produce sections. These go particularly well with trail mix since they don't spoil like fresh fruit.

Asparagus and Cashew Nuts

This healthy and satisfying snack is a unique way to get a serving of veggies. This dish also makes a satisfying accompaniment to a fish, chicken, turkey, or beef entrée.

INGREDIENTS | SERVES 2

2 tablespoons olive oil

2 tablespoons sesame oil

1 teaspoon minced gingerroot

½ pound asparagus, ends trimmed and cut into 2" pieces

1 teaspoon red pepper flakes

½ cup chopped cashews

Sesame Oil

Sesame oil is great for stir-frying. It has a high heat capacity and a relatively low smoke value so it cooks well under higher heat conditions. Additionally, sesame oil adds a nice Asian flavor to meals cooked with the oil.

1. Heat olive oil and sesame oil in a wok or large sauté pan over medium heat.

2. Add ginger and stir-fry until soft, about 5 minutes.

3. Add asparagus and red pepper flakes, and stir-fry for 3 minutes.

4. Add cashews. Cook until asparagus is tender, stirring frequently, about 5 minutes. Serve.

PER SERVING | Calories: 466 | Fat: 43 g | Protein: 8 g | Sodium: 9 mg | Fiber: 4 g | Carbohydrates: 17 g | Sugar: 4 g

Pistachio-Pumpkin Trail Mix

This trail mix is sure to satisfy someone who is always on the go. Feel free to add the types of nuts or fruit you like to make it your own personal trail mix.

INGREDIENTS | SERVES 4

½ cup pistachio nuts

½ cup pumpkin seeds

½ cup sunflower seeds

½ cup unsweetened coconut flakes

1 cup unsweetened dried cranberries or mulberries

Combine all ingredients. Store in an airtight container.

PER SERVING | Calories: 389 | Fat: 31 g | Protein: 17 g | Sodium: 12 mg | Fiber: 6 g | Carbohydrates: 17 g | Sugar: 4 g

Jicama Empanadas

These empanadas can be served fresh or they can be warmed in the oven at 250°F for 15 minutes or until heated through.

INGREDIENTS | SERVES 2

½ medium jicama
¼ cup fresh lime juice
¼ cup olive oil
1 teaspoon ground cumin, divided
½ teaspoon all-natural sea salt
1 cup walnuts
2 tablespoons green pumpkin seeds
1 tablespoon onion powder
½ medium clove garlic, minced
½ teaspoon ground cinnamon
½ tablespoon diced jalapeño pepper
1 tablespoon minced fresh oregano

1. Cut jicama into long, thin slices using a mandolin or grater.

2. Stir together lime juice, olive oil, ½ teaspoon cumin, and salt; brush oil mixture over jicama slices to coat lightly.

3. Process walnuts, pumpkin seeds, onion powder, garlic, remaining ½ teaspoon cumin, cinnamon, jalapeño, and oregano together in a food processer or blender.

4. Lay jicama slices flat. Place about 1 tablespoon filling onto half of each jicama slice. Fold other half of jicama slice over filling to create a pocket. Serve immediately.

PER SERVING │ Calories: 541 │ Fat: 51 g │ Protein: 11 g │ Sodium: 590 mg │ Fiber: 8 g │ Carbohydrates: 37 g │ Sugar: 7 g

Turkey Avocado Wraps

These wraps are simple and quick, yet absolutely delicious. They're great cut into smaller pieces for serving to little ones.

INGREDIENTS | SERVES 2

1 avocado
4 ounces sliced roasted turkey breast
2 tablespoons fresh lemon juice
½ cup diced tomatoes
1 teaspoon chopped fresh mint

Food Combining

When eating a snack or a meal, try to pay attention to the combinations of food that make up each dish. Besides enjoying a diversity of tastes, you're also helping each food group bring out the best in the others. Protein helps to repair muscles, carbohydrates aid in energy production, and fats promote healthy brain function. By combining all three groups within each meal, you can ensure that your body is getting all the nutrition it needs.

1. Slice avocado into thin strips.

2. Lay avocado slices over turkey and drizzle with lemon juice.

3. Top avocado with tomato and mint, wrap tightly, and enjoy.

PER SERVING | Calories: 358 | Fat: 18 g | Protein: 24 g | Sodium: 254 mg | Fiber: 8 g | Carbohydrates: 26 g | Sugar: 3 g

Floret Salad

This floret salad tastes even better when you allow it to sit overnight in the refrigerator so that the flavors can combine with each other.

INGREDIENTS | SERVES 2

⅔ cup cauliflower florets

⅔ cup broccoli florets

2 tablespoons chopped red onion

8 ounces uncured nitrate-free, sugar-free bacon, cooked and crumbled

1 tablespoon raw honey

¼ cup walnut oil

2 tablespoons cashew pieces

Broccoli: An Amazing Superfood

Broccoli is one of the healthiest vegetables you can eat. Ounce for ounce, broccoli has more vitamin C than an orange and as much calcium as a glass of milk. Broccoli is packed with fiber to promote digestive health and it is rich in vitamin A.

1. In a medium bowl, combine cauliflower, broccoli, red onion, and bacon.

2. In a small bowl, whisk together honey and walnut oil.

3. Combine honey mixture with vegetables and toss.

4. Top with cashews just before serving.

PER SERVING | Calories: 805 | Fat: 66 g | Protein: 45 g | Sodium: 2,743 mg | Fiber: 3 g | Carbohydrates: 18 g | Sugar: 11 g

Crunchy Fruit Salad

*When you're in the mood for a sweet treat, this crunchy salad will fulfill
that craving and replenish glycogen storage after workouts.*

INGREDIENTS | SERVES 4

½ pineapple, cubed

1 medium papaya, cubed

1 medium ripe banana, sliced

½ cup halved seedless grapes

1 tablespoon raw honey

¼ cup chopped cashews

¼ cup unsweetened coconut flakes

Combine all ingredients in a medium bowl and toss to mix.
Serve immediately or chill in refrigerator.

PER SERVING | Calories: 346 | Fat: 16 g | Protein: 6 g |
Sodium: 11 mg | Fiber: 6 g | Carbohydrates: 53 g | Sugar: 25 g

Seasonal Fruit

It is always best to eat foods that are native
to your area and in season. Imported fruits
have traveled long distances, so their fresh-
ness cannot be guaranteed. Your hunter-
gather ancestors did not have the luxury of
importing fruit from a neighboring area so
they only had access to foods that were in
season at the time of the hunt. Your diet
should change with the seasons.

Broccoli, Pine Nut, and Apple Salad

This quick little salad will tide you over until your next meal. The broccoli and apple taste great together, and the toasted pine nuts add a little bit of crunch.

INGREDIENTS | SERVES 2

¾ cup pine nuts
2 cups broccoli florets
2 cups diced green apples
Juice of 1 medium lemon

1. Toast pine nuts in a small frying pan until golden brown.

2. Mix broccoli and apples in a medium bowl. Add pine nuts and toss.

3. Squeeze lemon juice over salad and serve.

PER SERVING | Calories: 432 | Fat: 35 g | Protein: 10 g | Sodium: 33 mg | Fiber: 7 g | Carbohydrates: 28 g | Sugar: 15 g

CHAPTER 16

Smoothies and Juices

Blueberry Antioxidant Smoothie

Blueberries contain one of the highest antioxidant levels found in fruit. This smoothie refreshes you while fighting free-radical oxidation in your body.

INGREDIENTS | SERVES 1

1 cup blueberries

½ avocado

1 cup Homemade Almond Milk (see recipe in Chapter 10)

⅛ teaspoon ground nutmeg

4 ice cubes

Combine all ingredients in a blender and purée until smooth. Add additional ice cubes as needed for desired consistency.

PER SERVING | Calories: 289 | Fat: 24 g | Protein: 4 g | Sodium: 11 mg | Fiber: 11 g | Carbohydrates: 31 g | Sugar: 15 g

Very Cherry Vanilla Smoothie

Combining the unique flavors of cherries and vanilla with the smooth texture of delicious bananas and almond milk makes an incredible smoothie.

INGREDIENTS | SERVES 2

2 cups pitted dark sweet cherries

1 large banana

Pulp of 1 vanilla bean

1 cup Homemade Almond Milk (see recipe in Chapter 10)

1 teaspoon vanilla extract

1 cup ice, divided

1. Combine cherries, banana, vanilla bean pulp, almond milk, and vanilla extract in a blender with ½ cup ice and blend until thoroughly combined.

2. Add remaining ½ cup ice gradually while blending until desired consistency is reached.

PER SERVING | Calories: 200 | Fat: 5 g | Protein: 4 g | Sodium: 202 mg | Fiber: 6 g | Carbohydrates: 40 g | Sugar: 27 g

Where to Find Vanilla Beans

Vanilla beans can be found at your local grocery store. Whether the beans are stored in jars or plastic bags, whole beans can easily be located with the dried herbs or baking essentials. Slit the bean down the center with a sharp knife, open the skin, and reveal the pulp; this pulp is the ingredient referred to in the recipe lists in most cookbooks.

Tropical Smoothie

Mangoes are great to combat acidity and poor digestion and are often recommended for constipation. Mangoes contain phenols, a compound with powerful antioxidant and anti-cancer abilities.

INGREDIENTS | SERVES 2

1 small mango (about 1 cup diced)
½ small pineapple (about 1 cup diced)
1 very ripe large banana, sliced
1 cup unsweetened pineapple juice
½ cup coconut milk
1 teaspoon fresh lime juice

1. Peel and pit mango, then dice. Peel and core pineapple, then dice.

2. Arrange banana, mango, and pineapple in a single layer on a baking sheet.

3. Cover and freeze until fruit is frozen solid, about 2 hours.

4. Combine all ingredients in a blender. Cover and blend on high speed for 1 minute, or until smooth. Serve immediately.

PER SERVING | Calories: 370 | Fat: 15 g | Protein: 3 g | Sodium: 15 mg | Fiber: 6 g | Carbohydrates: 61 g | Sugar: 45 g

Pumpkin Spice Smoothie

If you're looking for an escape from the usual fruit smoothie, mix things up with this pumpkin pie in a glass. Raw ingredients and aromatic spices make this clean smoothie one of the most delicious and healthy dessert options around.

INGREDIENTS | SERVES 2

1 cup canned pumpkin

1 cup Homemade Almond Milk (see recipe in Chapter 10)

1 teaspoon ground cloves

1 teaspoon ground ginger

1 teaspoon ground cinnamon

2 cups ice, divided

1. Combine pumpkin, almond milk, and spices in a blender with 1 cup ice and blend until thoroughly combined.

2. Add remaining 1 cup ice gradually while blending until desired consistency is reached.

PER SERVING | Calories: 118 | Fat: 4 g | Protein: 3 g | Sodium: 227 mg | Fiber: 4 g | Carbohydrates: 19 g | Sugar: 5 g

Apple Pie Smoothie

Smooth, satisfying, aromatic, and absolutely mouthwatering, this smoothie packs all the healthiest ingredients into a tasty treat that will calm your craving for apple pie! It's not only a great guilt-free treat for you, but it's perfect for kids, too.

INGREDIENTS | SERVES 2

3 Granny Smith apples, cored

1 large banana

1 teaspoon ground cinnamon

1 teaspoon ground cloves

1 teaspoon ground nutmeg

1 teaspoon ground ginger

1 teaspoon vanilla extract

2 cups Homemade Almond Milk (see recipe in Chapter 10)

2 cups ice, divided

1. Preheat oven to 375°F.

2. Slice apples and layer in a shallow baking dish. Add enough water to cover bottom of baking dish about ½".

3. Bake for 20–30 minutes or until apples are fork-tender.

4. Combine cooked apples, banana, cinnamon, cloves, nutmeg, ginger, vanilla, and almond milk in a blender with ½ cup ice and blend until thoroughly combined.

5. Add remaining ice gradually while blending until desired consistency is reached.

PER SERVING | Calories: 279 | Fat: 9 g | Protein: 4 g | Sodium: 407 mg | Fiber: 8 g | Carbohydrates: 52 g | Sugar: 32 g

Banana Nut Blend Smoothie

*You can't replace waking up to the sweet aroma of fresh-baked
banana bread . . . until you taste this smoothie!*

INGREDIENTS | SERVES 2

¼ cup walnuts

1 cup Homemade Almond Milk (see recipe in Chapter 10), divided

1 cup chopped romaine lettuce

2 large bananas

1. Combine walnuts and ½ cup almond milk in a blender and blend until walnuts are completely emulsified.

2. Add romaine, bananas, and remaining almond milk while blending until desired texture is achieved.

PER SERVING | Calories: 228 | Fat: 11 g | Protein: 5 g | Sodium: 156 mg | Fiber: 5 g | Carbohydrates: 30 g | Sugar: 15 g

Walnuts and Antioxidants

When you think of antioxidant-rich foods, walnuts probably aren't your first thought, but just ¼ cup of walnuts provides almost 100 percent of your daily value of omega-3 fatty acids and is loaded with monounsaturated fats. Of the tree nuts, walnuts, chestnuts, and pecans carry the highest amount of antioxidants, which can prevent illness and reverse oxidative damage done by free radicals.

Mega Melon Smoothie

*The cool and lightly sweet refreshment that can only come from fresh melons
is bursting out of this smoothie. A great way to add fruit servings to your
day, this smoothie is the perfect treat on any hot afternoon.*

INGREDIENTS | SERVES 2

½ cantaloupe, cubed

½ honeydew melon, cubed

½ cup filtered water

1½ cups ice, divided

Hydrating Melons

Fruit smoothies are a tasty way to hydrate, and including melons in the mix makes for a truly satisfying treat. Packed with amazing amounts of vitamins and nutrients, these healthy fruits add tons of hydrating juices to any blended drink.

1. Combine cantaloupe, honeydew, water, and ½ cup ice in a blender and blend until thoroughly combined.

2. Add remaining ice while blending until desired consistency is achieved.

PER SERVING | Calories: 136 | Fat: 1 g | Protein: 3 g | Sodium: 67 mg | Fiber: 3 g | Carbohydrates: 34 g | Sugar: 31 g

Apricot-Banana Smoothie

The combination of apricots and banana make a delicious and refreshing smoothie.

INGREDIENTS | SERVES 1

3 large apricots, diced

1 large banana, diced

1 cup coconut milk

4 teaspoons raw honey

4 ice cubes

Combine all ingredients in a blender and blend until smooth and frosty. Add additional ice cubes if desired to reach preferred consistency.

PER SERVING | Calories: 544 | Fat: 30 g | Protein: 5 g | Sodium: 22 mg | Fiber: 9 g | Carbohydrates: 76 g | Sugar: 58 g

Apricots Are Quite Beneficial

Apricots are often overlooked as a fruit choice, but these little tangy fruit are an excellent source of potassium, iron, and vitamins A, C, and E. You could fulfill almost 50 percent of your vitamin A daily value with 3 apricots a day.

Stomach Soother Smoothie

Smoothies like this one help ease uncomfortable digestive symptoms. The ginger can soothe your stomach while satisfying your taste buds.

INGREDIENTS | SERVES 2

1 cup roughly chopped watercress

3 Gala apples, peeled and chopped

1 large banana, sliced

½" piece gingerroot, peeled

2 cups brewed red raspberry tea, divided

1. Combine watercress, apples, banana, ginger, and 1 cup tea in a blender and blend until thoroughly combined.

2. Add remaining tea as needed while blending until desired consistency is achieved.

PER SERVING | Calories: 260 | Fat: 1 g | Protein: 2 g | Sodium: 32 mg | Fiber: 5 g | Carbohydrates: 64 g | Sugar: 52 g

Beet the Bloat Smoothie

Beets are high in vitamins, minerals, and antioxidants that promote your body's ability to function optimally. By combining beets with apples, lemon, ginger, and green tea, you can fuel your body with the nutrients it needs while reducing bloat and gas.

INGREDIENTS | SERVES 3

1 cup roughly chopped beet greens

1 medium beet, roughly chopped

3 Gala apples, peeled and roughly chopped

½ medium lemon

¼" piece gingerroot, peeled

2 cups brewed green tea, divided

1. Combine beet greens, beet, apples, lemon, and ginger with 1 cup tea in a blender and blend until thoroughly combined.

2. Add remaining tea as needed while blending until desired consistency is achieved.

PER SERVING | Calories: 99 | Fat: 1 g | Protein: 1 g | Sodium: 75 mg | Fiber: 4 g | Carbohydrates: 23 g | Sugar: 17 g

Carrot Cleanser Smoothie

This simple recipe takes little time to make and tastes absolutely delicious. The carrots and lemon complement each other in this sweet and tangy smoothie.

INGREDIENTS | SERVES 2

1 cup roughly chopped spinach

4 medium carrots, peeled and roughly chopped

1 medium lemon, peeled

2 cups filtered water, divided

1. Combine spinach, carrots, lemon, and 1 cup water in a blender and blend until thoroughly combined.

2. Add remaining water while blending until desired texture is achieved.

PER SERVING | Calories: 62 | Fat: 0 g | Protein: 2 g | Sodium: 96 mg | Fiber: 4 g | Carbohydrates: 15 g | Sugar: 7 g

Carrots As Superfoods

Harnessing the powerful vitamins and minerals contained in carrots can help in many ways. The beta-carotene that gives carrots their vibrant color is not only important for eye health but is also a strong cancer-fighting antioxidant that protects cells against harmful free radicals. Carrots also lower the risk of heart disease, cancers, and type 2 diabetes and provide sound nutrition during pregnancy.

Vegetable Super Juice

*Add a generous dash of hot sauce to this juice for extra zip. It's
great on the rocks for a fast summer beverage.*

INGREDIENTS | SERVES 1

1 medium cucumber
6 large leaves romaine lettuce
4 medium stalks celery, including leaves
2 cups roughly chopped spinach
½ cup alfalfa sprouts
½ cup chopped fresh flat-leaf parsley

Sandy Spinach?

Spinach grows best in sandy soils, so it can be tough to rinse well. Rather than rinsing spinach through a colander, place it in a deep bowl and cover it with water. Gently toss to allow any sand or grit to fall to the bottom and lift the greens out.

1. Cut cucumber into pieces and process through a juicer according to the manufacturer's directions.

2. Wrap lettuce leaves around celery stalks and add to the feeding tube.

3. Add spinach, sprouts, and parsley.

4. Mix juice thoroughly before serving.

PER SERVING | Calories: 127 | Fat: 2 g | Protein: 8 g |
Sodium: 212 mg | Fiber: 4 g | Carbohydrates: 25 g | Sugar: 10 g

Cherry Cucumber Cooler

In addition to encouraging longer, stronger hair and nails, cherries hold a number of benefits for the eyes, including helping to prevent cataracts and macular degeneration.

INGREDIENTS | SERVES 1

1 medium cucumber, peeled
2 cups pitted sweet cherries
2 medium stalks celery, with leaves

All about Lutein

Cherries are rich in lutein, which is known to promote cardiovascular and eye health. Fat may help increase your body's absorption of lutein, so pair this with a few slices of avocado or a handful of nuts.

1. Process cucumber through an electronic juicer according to the manufacturer's directions.

2. Add cherries and process.

3. Add celery and process.

4. Stir or shake juice thoroughly to combine and serve over ice.

PER SERVING | Calories: 251 | Fat: 1 g | Protein: 6 g | Sodium: 70 mg | Fiber: 3 g | Carbohydrates: 62 g | Sugar: 45 g

Three-Grape Juice

When it comes to fruit juicing, little can compare with grapes. This trio provides a nice balance of flavor as the white and red grapes balance the more intense Concords.

INGREDIENTS | SERVES 1

1 cup Concord grapes
1 cup red globe grapes
1 cup white or green seedless grapes

Process grapes in an electronic juicer according to the manufacturer's directions. Serve alone or over ice.

PER SERVING | Calories: 312 | Fat: 1 g | Protein: 3 g | Sodium: 9 mg | Fiber: 3 g | Carbohydrates: 81 g | Sugar: 70 g

Great Grapes

Regarded in many cultures as "the queen of fruit," grapes are incredibly rich in phytonutrients, antioxidants, vitamins, and minerals and are a rich source of micronutrient minerals like copper, iron, and manganese.

Kiwi Apple Juice

Kiwifruit help remove excess sodium from the body, which can help you get rid of excess water and the bloat that comes along with it.

INGREDIENTS | SERVES 1

2 medium red apples, cored
3 medium kiwifruit

1. Process apples through an electronic juicer according to the manufacturer's directions.

2. Add kiwifruit and process.

3. Stir to mix juice and serve immediately.

PER SERVING | Calories: 244 | Fat: 1 g | Protein: 3 g | Sodium: 11 mg | Fiber: 15 g | Carbohydrates: 61 g | Sugar: 22 g

Peppermint Juice

In addition to great flavor, peppermint is a natural remedy for upset tummies.

INGREDIENTS | SERVES 3 (½-CUP SERVINGS)

½ cup fresh peppermint leaves
½ medium cucumber
½ cup bean sprouts
2 large leaves romaine lettuce

1. Process peppermint and cucumber through an electronic juicer according to the manufacturer's directions.

2. Add sprouts and lettuce and process. Stir to combine, and serve.

PER SERVING | Calories: 26 | Fat: 0 g | Protein: 2 g | Sodium: 9 mg | Fiber: 1 g | Carbohydrates: 5 g | Sugar: 1 g

CHAPTER 17

Kid-Friendly Recipes

Coconut Chicken Fingers

Anything but ordinary, these delicious chicken fingers are marinated in pineapple and coconut milk, and dressed in crunchy coconut flakes for a taste that's sure to be a hit with kids.

INGREDIENTS | SERVES 6

3 pounds boneless, skinless chicken tenders or breast strips (about 12 tenders)

½ cup coconut milk

½ cup unsweetened pineapple juice

2 cups unsweetened coconut flakes

Coconut Flakes Add Tons of Taste

If you're looking for a healthy sprinkling of fat to add to a favorite meal, reach no further than to a heaping helping of natural coconut flakes. Unsweetened varieties of coconut flakes are packed with tons of flavor without the added sugar. Toast them for added crunchiness, and use them as a delicious topping, a great addition to cookies, or even as a delicious sweet contrast to savory entrées.

1. Place tenders in a 1-gallon resealable plastic bag with coconut milk and pineapple juice, and marinate for 1–2 hours in refrigerator.

2. Preheat oven to 400°F. Line a baking sheet with foil and lightly grease with oil. Pour coconut flakes into a shallow dish.

3. Remove tenders from marinade and discard marinade. Place tenders in coconut flakes and turn to coat evenly. Arrange tenders on prepared baking sheet.

4. Bake for 20–25 minutes or until crispy.

PER SERVING | Calories: 670 | Fat: 34 g | Protein: 76 g | Sodium: 655 mg | Fiber: 6 g | Carbohydrates: 12 g | Sugar: 5 g

Yummy Meatballs

Almost everyone loves meatballs—and this gut-healthy recipe won't disappoint. Alone, or paired with sauce, these meatballs will be a favorite for the whole family.

INGREDIENTS | SERVES 6

2 tablespoons olive oil, divided
1 medium yellow onion, minced
½ medium red bell pepper, minced
½ medium green bell pepper, minced
2 teaspoons minced garlic
1 pound lean ground beef
1 teaspoon all-natural sea salt
1 teaspoon ground black pepper
1 large egg

1. Preheat oven to 350°F. Add 1 teaspoon olive oil to a large skillet over medium heat.

2. Add onion, peppers, and garlic to skillet; sauté until soft. Remove from heat and let cool.

3. In a large mixing bowl, combine ground beef, sautéed onion and peppers, salt, pepper, and egg; use your hands to mix well.

4. Form mixture into 24 (1½") balls.

5. Brush the rack of a roasting pan with remaining olive oil to coat lightly, and place over the roasting pan. Place meatballs 1" apart on rack.

6. Bake for 10 minutes. Turn, and bake for another 10 minutes, or until completely cooked through.

PER SERVING | Calories: 207 | Fat: 10 g | Protein: 24 g | Sodium: 448 mg | Fiber: 1 g | Carbohydrates: 3 g | Sugar: 2 g

"French Fry" Casserole

This recipe is a kid favorite that the whole family will love. Sweet potato fries, ground beef, and a simple slow-cooked cream sauce make a tasty weeknight meal. Serve with a salad or steamed green beans.

INGREDIENTS | SERVES 4

2 large sweet potatoes

1 pound lean ground beef

1 tablespoon coconut butter

½ medium Vidalia onion, finely diced

1 cup sliced button or cremini mushrooms

½ medium green bell pepper, diced

2 tablespoons arrowroot or tapioca powder

1⅓ cups coconut milk

½ teaspoon ground black pepper

Make-Ahead Sauce

You can make several batches of this cream sauce at the beginning of the week to make meals even easier to put together. Simply make a batch, pour into a glass jar with an airtight lid, and store in the refrigerator for up to 1 week.

1. Preheat oven to 375°F. Lightly grease a 4-quart slow cooker with oil.

2. Peel sweet potatoes and cut into fries. Place fries in a single layer on a baking sheet. Bake for 30 minutes, turning once.

3. In a large skillet over medium heat, cook the ground beef until browned, about 5–10 minutes. Drain off excess fat from beef and transfer meat to prepared slow cooker.

4. In a medium saucepan, melt coconut butter over medium heat. Add onion, mushrooms, and bell pepper; sauté for 3–5 minutes, until softened.

5. Mix arrowroot or tapioca powder with coconut milk and slowly add to cooked vegetables. Whisk together over medium heat until thickened, about 5–10 minutes.

6. Pour cream sauce with vegetables over ground beef in slow cooker. Sprinkle with pepper.

7. Top beef with sweet potato fries. Vent lid of slow cooker with a chopstick to prevent extra condensation on fries. Cook on high for 3 hours or on low for 5 hours.

PER SERVING | Calories: 224 | Fat: 11 g | Protein: 23 g | Sodium: 76 mg | Fiber: 1 g | Carbohydrates: 6 g | Sugar: 1 g

Stuffed Peppers

Peppers are chock-full of great vitamins and minerals that kids need. These peppers are so fun to eat, your children will request them as a regular part of the menu.

INGREDIENTS | SERVES 4

4 medium red bell peppers

2 tablespoons olive oil

3 medium cloves garlic, minced

1 medium yellow onion, chopped

1 pound ground chicken

2 medium green bell peppers, chopped

1 cup diced celery

1 cup sliced button or cremini mushrooms

2 tablespoons chili powder

1 tablespoon ground cumin

1 (28-ounce) can diced tomatoes

1 (6-ounce) can no-salt-added tomato paste

1. Cut off tops of red peppers and remove seeds and ribs, leaving peppers hollowed out and intact. Set aside.

2. In a large skillet, heat olive oil on medium; sauté garlic and onion for 2 minutes.

3. Add ground chicken and cook until browned, about 5–10 minutes.

4. Add bell peppers, celery, mushrooms, chili powder, and cumin, and continue cooking for 5 minutes.

5. Stuff mixture into red peppers and place in a 4-quart slow cooker.

6. Pour diced tomatoes and tomato paste over peppers. Cover and cook on high for 5 hours.

PER SERVING | Calories: 385 | Fat: 25 g | Protein: 23 g | Sodium: 159 mg | Fiber: 6 g | Carbohydrates: 17 g | Sugar: 9 g

Soft "Shell" Beef Tacos

*The romaine leaves used as shells in this recipe could also be placed
under the broiler until crispy, for use as a hard taco "shell."*

INGREDIENTS | SERVES 6

2 (16-ounce) jars mild or medium tomato-based salsa

2 tablespoons fresh lime juice

5 teaspoons chili powder

1½ pounds beef chuck pot roast, fat trimmed

12 large leaves romaine lettuce (for use as taco "shells")

3 cups shredded lettuce

1 avocado, diced

1. Spoon 1 cup salsa into a small bowl; set aside.

2. In a 4- to 6-quart slow cooker on low heat, combine remaining salsa with lime juice and chili powder. Add beef and cover. Cook for 10–12 hours, until tender.

3. Shred meat using 2 forks, and spoon into a serving bowl.

4. Lay out romaine leaves and place a small portion of slow-cooked beef on each.

5. Place shredded lettuce and diced avocado in separate small bowls for serving along with reserved salsa. Add toppings to tacos, wrap lettuce leaves tightly, and enjoy.

PER SERVING | Calories: 530 | Fat: 34 g | Protein: 37 g |
Sodium: 1,212 mg | Fiber: 10 g | Carbohydrates: 24 g | Sugar: 9 g

Turkey Lettuce Wraps

Turkey is a protein source that kids are sure to love. Although these wraps are a bit more complex to make, you can make a larger batch of the filling and serve it over salad at a later meal.

INGREDIENTS | SERVES 4

3 tablespoons walnut oil
3 medium shallots, chopped
1 (2") piece lemongrass, thinly sliced
½ teaspoon ground black pepper
1 pound ground turkey
⅓ cup fresh lime juice
2 tablespoons sesame oil
¼ cup coconut oil
½ cup thinly sliced fresh Thai basil leaves
8 large butter lettuce leaves

1. In a large skillet, heat walnut oil over medium heat.

2. Add shallots, lemongrass, and pepper. Cook until shallots soften, about 4 minutes.

3. Add ground turkey and stir frequently until cooked through, approximately 8–10 minutes.

4. Add lime juice, sesame oil, and coconut oil and cook for 1 minute. Turn off heat and mix in basil.

5. Wrap mixture in lettuce leaves and serve.

PER SERVING | Calories: 483 | Fat: 37 g | Protein: 33 g | Sodium: 300 mg | Fiber: 2 g | Carbohydrates: 12 g | Sugar: 1 g

Almond Butter Celery Sticks

Getting your kids to eat their veggies is no chore with these "ants on a log." The sweetness of smooth almond butter and chewy raisins atop the crispy crunch of celery make it a noisy favorite.

INGREDIENTS | SERVES 4

4 large stalks celery
½ cup almond butter
¼ cup unsweetened raisins

Combine Texture and Flavor

Even the pickiest of eaters normally enjoy celery topped with nut butter. The sweet almond butter is a tasty treat atop the crunchy celery sticks. With protein from the almond butter, rich carbohydrates, and hydrating water in the celery, it's got a plethora of nutritional benefits.

1. Cut off ends and tops of celery. Cut celery stalks in half crosswise.

2. Fill hollow of stalks with almond butter.

3. Line raisins on top of almond butter.

PER SERVING │ Calories: 164 │ Fat: 8 g │ Protein: 3 g │ Sodium: 36 mg │ Fiber: 2 g │ Carbohydrates: 22 g │ Sugar: 16 g

Mashed Potatoes and Cauliflower

Rather than using only potatoes in your traditional mashed potatoes, you could always use this recipe instead. The blend of herbs and spices makes the dish extra-flavorful.

INGREDIENTS | SERVES 6

1 pound Idaho potatoes, peeled and cubed

1 pound cauliflower florets

2 teaspoons garlic powder

1 teaspoon onion powder

1 teaspoon all-natural sea salt

1 teaspoon ground black pepper

2 cups Homemade Almond Milk (see recipe in Chapter 10)

1 tablespoon chopped green onion

Sneak in the Nutrition

While potatoes have loads of nutrition and tons of health benefits, there are healthy alternatives that offer different nutritional value. Adding cauliflower to your pot of boiling potatoes will result in a creamy bowl of mashed delight that's not far off from the original. The added bonus to the lower calorie load of the dish is a better variety of vitamins and minerals and the same great taste.

1. In a large pot over medium heat, bring potato cubes to a boil, reduce heat to low, and simmer for 10 minutes.

2. Add cauliflower to pot and simmer for an additional 10 minutes, or until cauliflower is fork-tender.

3. Remove pot from heat, drain, and transfer potatoes and cauliflower to a large bowl. Season with garlic powder, onion powder, salt, and pepper.

4. Mash or beat potatoes and cauliflower, adding almond milk ¼ cup at a time until desired texture is achieved.

5. Transfer to serving bowl, sprinkle green onions on top, and serve hot.

PER SERVING | Calories: 89 | Fat: 0 g | Protein: 3 g | Sodium: 481 mg | Fiber: 4 g | Carbohydrates: 17 g | Sugar: 2 g

Chicken Nuggets

These chicken nuggets are fantastic for kids and adults. Serve them with a salad or sweet potato fries.

1. Preheat oven to 475°F.

2. In small bowl, mix olive oil, garlic, and pepper.

3. Place chicken in a shallow dish. Pour marinade over chicken and marinate for 30 minutes in refrigerator.

4. Place almond flour in a shallow bowl. Remove chicken from marinade and dredge in almond flour to coat.

5. Bake for 10 minutes or until brown, turning halfway through baking time to brown both sides evenly. Serve.

PER SERVING | Calories: 369 | Fat: 28 g | Protein: 20 g | Sodium: 2 mg | Fiber: 2 g | Carbohydrates: 12 g | Sugar: 0 g

Chocolate Chip Cookies

These cookies are a twist on the classic favorite. You can allow your children to indulge in some comfort food while also protecting their gut health.

INGREDIENTS | SERVES 12

1 cup sunflower seed butter
½ cup raw honey
1 large egg
2 teaspoons baking soda
1⅓ cups almond meal
¾ cup cacao nibs

1. Preheat oven to 350°F. Line a baking sheet with parchment paper.

2. In the bowl of a mixer, blend sunflower butter and honey until well mixed.

3. Add egg and baking soda and mix for 2 minutes.

4. Add almond meal and mix, then add cacao nibs and stir.

5. Spoon dough by rounded tablespoonsful onto prepared baking sheet and bake for 10–15 minutes, until lightly browned.

6. Remove to wire rack and let cool completely.

PER SERVING | Calories: 286 | Fat: 14 g | Protein: 4 g | Sodium: 12 mg | Fiber: 2 g | Carbohydrates: 39 g | Sugar: 12 g

Chocolate Bars

Your kids will be thrilled when they see these chocolate bars in their lunchboxes. These bars are quick to whip up and quick to eat. You can vary the amount of honey depending on your desired sweetness level.

INGREDIENTS | SERVES 8

1 tablespoon raw honey
¼ cup coconut oil
¼ cup ground almonds
¼ cup ground hazelnuts
¼ cup sunflower seeds
¼ cup cacao powder
¾ cup unsweetened coconut flakes

1. Melt honey and coconut oil in a small saucepan over medium heat.

2. In a medium mixing bowl, combine almonds, hazelnuts, sunflower seeds, cacao powder, and coconut. Mix thoroughly.

3. Add honey mixture to bowl and mix well.

4. Pour dough into an 8" × 8" dish and place in freezer until firm, about 10 minutes.

5. Cut into squares and enjoy.

PER SERVING | Calories: 154 | Fat: 15 g | Protein: 2 g | Sodium: 2 mg | Fiber: 2 g | Carbohydrates: 5 g | Sugar: 3 g

Banana Sorbet

Ice cream and store-bought sorbets can be packed with sugar and impossible-to-pronounce ingredients. This recipe calls for only 4 ingredients, and makes for a sweet treat your kids will ask for time and time again.

INGREDIENTS | SERVES 4

4 large frozen bananas (peeled and bagged prior to freezing)
2 teaspoons vanilla extract
1 teaspoon ground nutmeg
1 teaspoon raw honey

Simplicity Can Be Key

When creating delicious and nutritious meals that will appeal to kids, there is one key point to remember: Keep it simple. Because children haven't had more than a few short years of eating different foods, they may be hesitant to eat something that combines too many flavors—even if it's just one flavor they dislike among a ton they love. Keep it limited to a handful of ingredients, and add more little by little as they grow up.

1. In a high-speed blender, purée bananas and vanilla.

2. While blending, add nutmeg and honey and purée until smooth.

3. Pour banana mixture into small serving cups or bowls and freeze for 10 minutes before serving.

PER SERVING | Calories: 119 | Fat: 0 g | Protein: 1 g | Sodium: 2 mg | Fiber: 4 g | Carbohydrates: 29 g | Sugar: 16 g

Slow-Cooked Sloppy Joeys

Serve these fun Sloppy Joeys over mashed cauliflower, turnips, or winter squash.

INGREDIENTS | SERVES 4

1 pound lean ground beef
1 (6-ounce can) tomato paste
2 tablespoons raw honey
1 tablespoon dried onion flakes
1 tablespoon ground paprika
1 teaspoon ground cumin
1 teaspoon fresh lemon juice
½ teaspoon garlic powder
¼ teaspoon dry mustard
¼ teaspoon celery seed
¼ teaspoon ground black pepper
1 cup warm filtered water
1 teaspoon almond meal

1. Sauté meat in a frying pan for 5 to 10 minutes, or until browned. Drain juices.

2. Add all ingredients to a 4-quart slow cooker and stir to mix and break up the ground meat.

3. Cover and cook on low for 6–7 hours or on high for 3–5 hours. Serve warm.

PER SERVING | Calories: 234 | Fat: 6 g | Protein: 26 g | Sodium: 414 mg | Fiber: 3 g | Carbohydrates: 18 g | Sugar: 14 g

Sweet Fruit Bake

This is a great fruit combination. When mixed with the lemon juice, it can be presented at any time without fear of it turning brown.

INGREDIENTS | SERVES 8

2 cups blueberries
2 cups quartered strawberries
2 cups sliced peaches
2 cups sliced Green Anjou pears
1 tablespoon fresh lemon juice
1 teaspoon lemon zest

1. Preheat oven to 350°F. Grease a 9" × 13" baking dish.

2. In a large mixing bowl, toss fruit with lemon juice and lemon zest.

3. Pour fruit into prepared baking dish and bake for 25–35 minutes, or until all fruit is tender. Serve warm.

PER SERVING | Calories: 85 | Fat: 0 g | Protein: 1 g | Sodium: 2 mg | Fiber: 3 g | Carbohydrates: 22 g | Sugar: 17 g

Picking Your Pear

Green Anjou pears have a mellow, citrus-y flavor and a juicy texture. If you're looking for a little more kick, replace the Green Anjou pear with a Red Anjour pear, which has hints of sweet spice instead of citrus.

Banana-Coconut Muffins

These banana muffins made with coconut flour are a great wheat-free alternative to traditional muffins.

INGREDIENTS | SERVES 12

½ cup coconut flour
¼ teaspoon all-natural sea salt
½ teaspoon baking powder
4 large eggs
¼ cup coconut oil
¼ cup raw honey
2 large ripe bananas, mashed
½ cup walnuts

1. Preheat oven to 350°F. Grease a 12-cup muffin pan.

2. Mix together all ingredients. Scoop batter into prepared muffin pan, filling cups ⅔ full.

3. Bake for 15 minutes, or until golden brown. Serve warm.

PER SERVING | Calories: 151 | Fat: 9 g | Protein: 4 g | Sodium: 92 mg | Fiber: 3 g | Carbohydrates: 15 g | Sugar: 9 g

Coconut Flour

Coconut flour is dehydrated coconut meat that has had most of the oil removed and been ground to a powdery consistency. It is not good for thickening sauces, but it works very well for baking. It is gluten-free and high in protein.

Strawberry Breakfast Smoothie

A deliciously rich strawberry banana smoothie will be your kids' favorite breakfast after just one taste.

INGREDIENTS | SERVES 3 (1-CUP
SERVINGS)

1 cup roughly chopped romaine lettuce

2 pints strawberries, hulled

2 large bananas

1 cup strawberry kefir

1 cup ice

1. Combine romaine, strawberries, bananas, and kefir in a blender and blend until thoroughly combined.

2. Add ice as needed while blending until desired consistency is achieved.

PER SERVING | Calories: 226 | Fat: 3 g | Protein: 5 g | Sodium: 142 mg | Fiber: 8 g | Carbohydrates: 47 g | Sugar: 30 g

Chocolate Dream Smoothie

Your little ones (and their adult counterparts) will fall for the deliciously rich flavors of this recipe.

INGREDIENTS | SERVES 3 (1-CUP SERVINGS)

1 cup roughly chopped spinach

2 tablespoons carob powder

3 large bananas

2 cups Homemade Almond Milk (see recipe in Chapter 10), divided

1 cup ice

1. Combine spinach, carob powder, bananas, and 1 cup almond milk in a blender and blend until thoroughly combined.

2. Add remaining almond milk and ice as needed while blending until desired consistency is achieved.

PER SERVING | Calories: 173 | Fat: 6 g | Protein: 20 g | Sodium: 22 mg | Fiber: 5 g | Carbohydrates: 34 g | Sugar: 17 g

Green Goblin Juice

This juice has a pronounced grape flavor and a great green color.
They'll never suspect there's spinach in there!

INGREDIENTS | SERVES 2 (1-CUP SERVINGS)

2 cups white or green seedless grapes

½ cup roughly chopped spinach

1 cup filtered water

1. Process grapes through an electronic juicer according to the manufacturer's directions.

2. Add spinach and process.

3. Add water and mix.

PER SERVING | Calories: 63 | Fat: 0 g | Protein: 1 g | Sodium: 8 mg | Fiber: 1 g | Carbohydrates: 16 g | Sugar: 15 g

Orangeberry Juice

This juice contains an array of nutrients to give kids energy, making it an excellent addition to breakfast.

INGREDIENTS | SERVES 3 (½-CUP SERVINGS)

1 cup raspberries
2 oranges
2 pitted nectarines

Oranges and Calcium

Orange-based juice is important for kids because the calcium it contains helps to build strong bones. A medium-sized orange has 52 mg of calcium.

1. Process raspberries and oranges through an electronic juicer according to the manufacturer's directions.

2. Add nectarines and process.

3. Whisk or shake juice and serve.

PER SERVING | Calories: 121 | Fat: 1 g | Protein: 3 g | Sodium: 0 mg | Fiber: 7 g | Carbohydrates: 29 g | Sugar: 21 g

Desserts and Sweets

Chia Pudding

Chia seeds are a nutritional powerhouse. A single ounce of chia seeds contains 11 g of fiber—almost half your needs for the entire day. The tiny seeds are also loaded with protein and omega-3 fatty acids as well as a combination of vitamins and minerals.

INGREDIENTS | SERVES 4

1 cup coconut milk

1 cup Homemade Almond Milk (see recipe in Chapter 10)

1 teaspoon vanilla extract

1 tablespoon unsweetened cocoa powder

1 tablespoon raw honey

2 tablespoons unsweetened coconut flakes

½ cup chia seeds

¼ cup blackberries

1. Blend coconut milk, almond milk, vanilla extract, cocoa powder, and honey in blender.

2. Add coconut flakes and chia seeds to mixture and stir until evenly dispersed. Cover and refrigerate for 8 hours. Spoon into serving bowls and top with blackberries.

PER SERVING | Calories: 256 | Fat: 23 g | Protein: 5 g | Sodium: 12 mg | Fiber: 8 g | Carbohydrates: 16 g | Sugar: 7 g

Poached Pears and Raspberries

You can substitute other fruit, such as apples, peaches, apricots, or plums, in this recipe.

INGREDIENTS | SERVES 4

1 cup unsweetened white grape juice
¼ cup unsweetened apple juice
1 teaspoon ground cinnamon
1 teaspoon ground nutmeg
4 large Bartlett pears
½ cup raspberries
2 tablespoons orange zest

1. Combine juices in a bowl, then slowly stir in cinnamon and nutmeg.

2. Peel pears, leaving stems intact, and core from the bottom.

3. Stand pears in a deep skillet. Slowly add juice mixture to skillet and bring to a simmer over medium heat (do not boil). Cover and simmer for 30 minutes until tender.

4. Place pears upright on individual serving plates and spoon juice over the top. Garnish with raspberries and orange zest, or purée berries with zest in a blender and pour over pears.

PER SERVING │ Calories: 163 │ Fat: 1 g │ Protein: 1 g │ Sodium: 10 mg │ Fiber: 6 g │ Carbohydrates: 40 g │ Sugar: 29 g

Blueberry Pie

*Scrumptious blueberry pie gets a healthy makeover in this recipe. Skip the
sugar and let the sweetness of the blueberries speak for itself.*

INGREDIENTS | SERVES 8

3 dates, pitted
⅔ cup coconut milk
3 cups blueberries
1 prepared Clean Pie Crust (see recipe in
this chapter)

1. In a blender, combine dates and coconut milk, and blend until emulsified and thickened.

2. In a small saucepan over medium heat, bring date mixture to a boil. Reduce heat, add blueberries, and simmer for 5 minutes.

3. Remove saucepan from heat and let cool for 5–10 minutes.

4. Pour blueberry mixture into prepared pie shell. Let set in refrigerator for at least 3 hours, or overnight.

PER SERVING | Calories: 159 | Fat: 9 g | Protein: 2 g |
Sodium: 76 mg | Fiber: 2 g | Carbohydrates: 20 g | Sugar: 8 g

Walnut Pecan Brownies with Raspberry Sauce

These brownies are ideal with a cream berry sauce spread on the top. You can substitute other types of berries or fruit in place of the raspberries.

INGREDIENTS | SERVES 6

2 cups walnuts

2 cups pecans

1 cup dried dates

½ cup carob powder

½ tablespoon ground cinnamon

¼ cup raw honey

½ teaspoon all-natural sea salt

½ cup melted coconut oil

1 recipe Raspberry Sauce (see recipe in this chapter)

1. Blend walnuts and pecans in a food processor until they are roughly chopped. Do not overprocess.

2. Add dates, carob powder, cinnamon, honey, salt, and melted coconut oil and process until well mixed.

3. Press batter into a 8" × 8" square pan. Pour Raspberry Sauce evenly on top.

4. Place pan in freezer for about 1 hour, until hardened. Slice into squares.

PER SERVING | Calories: 707 | Fat: 61 g | Protein: 10 g | Sodium: 198 mg | Fiber: 11 g | Carbohydrates: 39 g | Sugar: 31 g

Raspberry Sauce

This is a creamy berry sauce that tastes great on brownies or ice cream or as a dressing for fruit salad. You can substitute other types of berries or fruit in place of the raspberries.

INGREDIENTS | MAKES 2 CUPS (½-CUP SERVINGS)

2 cups raspberries
1 cup young coconut meat
¼ cup young coconut water

In a blender or food processor, blend raspberries with coconut meat and water until smooth.

PER SERVING | Calories: 54 | Fat: 1 g | Protein: 1 g | Sodium: 16 mg | Fiber: 4 g | Carbohydrates: 12 g | Sugar: 7 g

Fruit Pops

Made with love and natural ingredients, these pops are healthier and more nutritious than commercially prepared popsicles, and you're able to control the ingredients and amounts to tailor them specifically to your likes and dislikes.

INGREDIENTS | SERVES 6

1 large banana
1 cup hulled strawberries
1½ cups fresh-squeezed orange juice

1. In a high-speed blender, combine all ingredients.

2. Pour fruit mixture into 6 individual pop molds. Freeze overnight.

3. Remove pops by running the pop molds under warm water until pops release.

PER SERVING | Calories: 56 | Fat: 0 g | Protein: 1 g | Sodium: 1 mg | Fiber: 1 g | Carbohydrates: 14 g | Sugar: 9 g

Frozen Delights

There's something whimsical about food on a stick. Taking into consideration that kids love sweetness, frozen treats, and anything they can hold in one hand and enjoy, pops have it all wrapped up in a single delicious serving.

Cherry Chocolate Pudding

This smooth and creamy dessert is made with real chocolate. You can substitute macadamia nuts in place of the young coconut. If cherries are out of season, frozen cherries will work well.

INGREDIENTS | SERVES 4

¼ cup roughly chopped dates
¾ cup young coconut meat
½ cup young coconut water
2 tablespoons cacao powder
1 cup pitted dark cherries

1. In a blender or food processor, combine dates, coconut meat and water, and cacao powder; blend well.

2. Add cherries and briefly pulse until mixed in but still chunky. Pour into bowls and serve.

PER SERVING | Calories: 130 | Fat: 3 g | Protein: 2 g | Sodium: 32 mg | Fiber: 3 g | Carbohydrates: 20 g | Sugar: 14 g

Fruit Kebabs

Kebabs are just plain fun. When your kids need a snack, give them these fruit kebabs to keep them full—and entertained!

INGREDIENTS | SERVES 4

1 cup green seedless grapes
1 cup pineapple chunks
1 cup halved strawberries
1 cup red seedless grapes
1 cup blueberries

1. Thread fruit onto 4 skewers, alternating types in order listed and condensing firmly. Serve.

2. If serving children under 7, do not skewer fruit; serve fruit in small serving bowls instead.

PER SERVING | Calories: 105 | Fat: 0 g | Protein: 1 g | Sodium: 3 mg | Fiber: 3 g | Carbohydrates: 27 g | Sugar: 21 g

Banana Bread

This banana bread is a nice dessert or breakfast treat. You can intensify the flavor by adding more ripe bananas.

INGREDIENTS | SERVES 8

1¼ cups almond meal

2 teaspoons baking powder

¼ teaspoon baking soda

½ cup fruit purée of your choice

¼ teaspoon ground cinnamon

½ teaspoon vanilla extract

2 large eggs

3 large ripe bananas, mashed

¼ cup flaxseed flour

½ cup chopped walnuts

½ cup unsweetened coconut flakes

Bananas

Bananas are a great fruit, but they do raise your blood sugar significantly. In order to maximize the influx of sugar, these are always best when eaten after a workout.

1. Preheat oven to 350°F. Spray a 9" × 5" loaf pan with cooking spray.

2. In a large bowl, combine almond meal, baking powder, baking soda, fruit purée, cinnamon, and vanilla.

3. Add eggs, banana, and flaxseed flour. Mix well.

4. Fold walnuts and coconut flakes into batter. Pour batter into prepared pan.

5. Bake for 45 minutes. Cool in pan for 5 minutes, then transfer to wire rack to cool completely.

PER SERVING | Calories: 254 | Fat: 10 g | Protein: 6 g | Sodium: 65 mg | Fiber: 6 g | Carbohydrates: 39 g | Sugar: 7 g

Pumpkin Pudding

This pumpkin pudding is a great dessert for the holidays. If you're feeding a crowd, try serving it alongside Pecan Pie or Blueberry Pie (see recipes in this chapter).

INGREDIENTS | SERVES 8

2 large eggs
1 teaspoon ground cinnamon
½ teaspoon ground nutmeg
½ teaspoon ground cloves
½ teaspoon ground ginger
1 (15-ounce) can pumpkin
1 (14-ounce) can coconut milk
½ cup crushed pecans

Pumpkin: Not Just for Halloween

Many people write pumpkin off as just another Halloween decoration, but the fruit—which is actually technically a berry—is loaded with beneficial nutrients, including fiber, magnesium, calcium, and vitamins A, C, and E.

1. Preheat oven to 375°F. Grease an 8" × 8" square baking pan.

2. Whisk eggs in a medium bowl. Add spices and whisk again.

3. Add pumpkin and coconut milk and mix thoroughly.

4. Pour batter into prepared pan and top with pecans.

5. Bake for 45 minutes. Serve warm.

PER SERVING | Calories: 200 | Fat: 18 g | Protein: 4 g | Sodium: 26 mg | Fiber: 3 g | Carbohydrates: 9 g | Sugar: 4 g

Pecan Pie

Pecan pie is normally dismissed from a healthy plate because of its ingredients and nutritional content (or the lack thereof). This clean version, however, is great for gut health! It's so simple and extraordinarily tasty that you'll wonder why anyone ever made it any other way.

INGREDIENTS | SERVES 8

4 cups pecans, divided

¾ cup coconut oil

1 cup raw honey

1½ cups pitted dates

1 teaspoon ground nutmeg

1 teaspoon ground cinnamon

1 teaspoon ground cloves

1 prepared Clean Pie Crust (see recipe in this chapter)

1. In a food processor or blender, process 3 cups pecans, coconut oil, honey, and dates until thickened. Transfer to a large mixing bowl and add nutmeg, cinnamon, and cloves; blend well.

2. Pour pecan mixture into pie shell. Top with remaining pecans, pressing them lightly into pie filling. Let pie set in the refrigerator for 3–4 hours before serving.

PER SERVING | Calories: 865 | Fat: 65 g | Protein: 7 g | Sodium: 76 mg | Fiber: 9 g | Carbohydrates: 77 g | Sugar: 58 g

Pecan Pie Gets a Clean Makeover

Pecans are an amazing source of protein and healthy fats, and combining them with other fresh natural ingredients in this pie delivers the same great taste as traditional, but not-so-healthy, versions. Healthy, packed with benefits for the body and the brain, and amazingly delicious, this is a pie that hits the spot—from the crust to the filling to the topping!

Clean Pie Crust

Forget store-bought pie crusts! This is a simple and quick no-bake pie crust that's crunchy and delicious. Use it for the other pies in this chapter or any pie that does not require baking.

INGREDIENTS | MAKES 1 PIE CRUST (8 SERVINGS)

1 cup plus 2 tablespoons coconut oil, divided

4 cups macadamia nuts

5 dates, pitted

1. Coat a 9" pie dish with 2 tablespoons coconut oil.

2. Combine remaining 1 cup coconut oil with nuts and dates in a food processor and process until smooth.

3. Spoon mixture into prepared pan and press to ¼" thickness. Fill crust and let set according to directions in pie recipe.

PER SERVING | Calories: 760 | Fat: 81 g | Protein: 5 g | Sodium: 3 mg | Fiber: 6 g | Carbohydrates: 13 g | Sugar: 6 g

Tropical Paradise Pie

Traditional pineapple upside-down cake is no competition for this delicious recipe. Packed with crushed pineapple and fresh cherries, tossed in a creamy coconut sauce, and layered in a homemade crunchy pie crust, this is one recipe that is a delicious stretch from the ordinary. Plus, it's as much a visual treat as a culinary one.

INGREDIENTS | SERVES 8

3 dates, pitted
⅔ cup coconut milk
1 tablespoon raw honey
4 cups crushed pineapple
½ cup pitted dark cherries
1 prepared Clean Pie Crust (see recipe in this chapter)

1. In a blender, combine dates and coconut milk, and blend until emulsified and thickened.

2. In a medium saucepan over medium heat, bring date mixture to a boil. Reduce heat to a simmer and add honey, pineapple, and cherries; simmer for 5 minutes.

3. Remove saucepan from heat and let cool for 5–10 minutes.

4. Pour pineapple mixture into prepared pie shell. Let set in refrigerator for at least 3 hours, or overnight.

PER SERVING │ Calories: 941 │ Fat: 90 g │ Protein: 7 g │ Sodium: 79 mg │ Fiber: 8 g │ Carbohydrates: 37 g │ Sugar: 19 g

Almond Butter Cookies

Almond cookies are a great snack. They provide you with essential omega-6 and omega-3 fatty acids and are a good source of vitamin E.

INGREDIENTS | SERVES 12

1 cup almond butter

1 large egg white

2 tablespoons unsweetened applesauce

2 tablespoons unsweetened coconut flakes

1 tablespoon cacao powder

1. Preheat oven to 375°F.

2. Beat all ingredients together to form a thick batter.

3. Place dough by the tablespoonful onto an ungreased cookie sheet. Bake for 10–12 minutes or until lightly brown on top.

PER SERVING | Calories: 151 | Fat: 14 g | Protein: 4 g | Sodium: 9 mg | Fiber: 2 g | Carbohydrates: 6 g | Sugar: 0 g

Strawberries with Coconut Shortcake

This is like classic strawberry shortcake—without as much refined sugar!
This version of the classic dessert is much easier to digest.

INGREDIENTS | SERVES 8

⅓ cup melted coconut oil
6 large eggs
¼ cup coconut sugar
½ teaspoon all-natural sea salt
½ teaspoon vanilla extract
½ cup coconut flour
½ teaspoon baking soda
2 pounds strawberries, sliced
1 cup coconut cream, divided

1. Preheat oven to 400°F. Grease and flour a 12-cup muffin pan.

2. In a medium bowl, mix coconut oil, eggs, sugar, salt, and vanilla.

3. Add coconut flour and baking soda and stir to make a batter. Pour into prepared muffin pan, filling each cup about halfway.

4. Bake for about 15 minutes, or until golden brown. Remove shortcakes from pan and let cool on a wire rack for 10–15 minutes.

5. Cut shortcakes in half. Spoon ¼ cup strawberries on bottom halves and replace shortcake tops. Top shortcakes with 2 tablespoons coconut cream and a few more strawberry slices. Serve.

PER SERVING | Calories: 355 | Fat: 20 g | Protein: 7 g |
Sodium: 289 mg | Fiber: 5 g | Carbohydrates: 40 g | Sugar: 13 g

Chocolate Coconut Milk Balls

These coconut milk balls are not as creamy as ice cream, but they are a nice alternative. You can change the flavor by changing the type of fruit purée that you use in the recipe.

INGREDIENTS | SERVES 10

¾ cup cacao powder

6 tablespoons fresh fruit purée of your choice, such as raspberry, blueberry, or strawberry

6 tablespoons coconut oil

6 tablespoons coconut milk

3 tablespoons unsweetened shredded coconut

2 tablespoons cacao nibs

1 large ripe banana

1. Combine all ingredients in a food processor and process until very smooth.

2. Add water if the consistency is not fluid.

3. Pour into ice-cube trays and freeze until set.

PER SERVING | Calories: 149 | Fat: 13 g | Protein: 2 g | Sodium: 4 mg | Fiber: 4 g | Carbohydrates: 11 g | Sugar: 3 g

Coconut

Coconut has many great properties. This recipe uses all the edible parts of the coconut—the meat, oil, and milk. You will receive high fiber, vitamin, and mineral content as well as skin benefits from consumption of coconut.

Baked Bananas

This healthy dessert is sure to be a favorite. Make in bulk and use to spread on pancakes or waffles.

INGREDIENTS | SERVES 4

4 small bananas
½ teaspoon orange zest
¼ cup fruit purée
½ tablespoon raw honey
1 tablespoon fresh lemon juice
⅛ teaspoon ground cinnamon
⅛ teaspoon ground nutmeg
1 tablespoon melted coconut oil
1 tablespoon cacao nibs

1. Preheat oven to 350°F.

2. Cut each banana in half lengthwise and then cut each half across to make 8 pieces. Arrange banana pieces in a small baking pan.

3. Sprinkle evenly with orange zest, fruit purée, honey, lemon juice, cinnamon, nutmeg, and coconut oil.

4. Bake uncovered for 35–40 minutes, basting after 15 minutes with liquid in dish.

5. Sprinkle with cacao nibs before serving.

PER SERVING | Calories: 200 | Fat: 5 g | Protein: 2 g | Sodium: 2 mg | Fiber: 5 g | Carbohydrates: 41 g | Sugar: 16 g

Whipped Cream

This is a great clean version of whipped topping. With only 3 delicious ingredients whipped together for a delightfully light and sweet treat, this is a simple and delicious topping for any of your favorite desserts.

INGREDIENTS | SERVES 8 (¼-CUP SERVINGS)

2 (14-ounce) cans coconut milk
1½ tablespoons raw honey
1½ tablespoons vanilla extract

Yes, You Can Still Enjoy Whipped Cream!

Clean eating is all about living healthier, not about deprivation. By using healthy natural ingredients to create more nutritious versions of your favorite foods, you can still indulge.

1. Combine all ingredients in a mixing bowl. Using a high-speed blender, whip ingredients until thickened.

2. Refrigerate overnight and serve.

PER SERVING | Calories: 219 | Fat: 22 g | Protein: 2 g | Sodium: 14 mg | Fiber: 0 g | Carbohydrates: 6 g | Sugar: 3 g

Appendix A: Additional Resources

Austin UltraHealth, Amy Myers, MD

5656 Bee Caves Road
Suite D 203
Austin, TX 78746
(512) 383-5343
www.amymyersmd.com
Dr. Amy Myers is a functional medicine doctor who understands individuality in genetics and physiology. Her treatment approach focuses on getting to the root cause of your symptoms and treating you as an individual.

Chris Kresser, LAc

Chriskresser.com
Chris Kresser is a licensed acupuncturist and an integrative medicine practitioner. He works directly with patients to correct chronic health problems without the use of unnecessary medications.

Environmental Working Group

1436 U Street NW
Suite 100
Washington, DC 20009
(202) 667-6982
www.ewg.org
The EWG is an organization that empowers people to live healthier lives in a healthier environment by providing information about the latest scientific research.

The Institute for Functional Medicine

505 S. 336th Street
Suite 500
Federal Way, WA 98003
1-800-228-0622
www.functionalmedicine.org
The goal of the Institute for Functional Medicine is to reverse chronic disease and advance knowledge by providing information and education about functional medicine.

The UltraWellness Center

Dr. Mark Hyman
55 Pittsfield Road
Suite 9
Lenox Commons, Lenox, MA 01240
(413) 637-9991
www.ultrawellnesscenter.com
Dr. Mark Hyman is one of the leaders in functional medicine. He founded the UltraWellness Center in Lenox, Massachusetts, and has authored several books.

The Weston A. Price Foundation

PMB 106-380
4200 Wisconsin Avenue NW
Washington, DC 20016
(202) 363-4394
www.westonaprice.org
The Weston A. Price Foundation is a nonprofit organization dedicated to informing the public

about the importance of a nutrient-dense, real-foods diet.

WholeHealth Chicago

The Center for Integrative Medicine
2522 N. Lincoln Avenue
Chicago, IL 60614
(773) 296-6700
Wholehealthchicago.com
The practitioners at WholeHealth Chicago rely on evidence-based medicine and an individualized treatment approach to transform chronic illness by addressing physical, spiritual, and emotional aspects.

Women to Women

3 Marina Road
Yarmouth, ME 04096
(207) 846-6163
www.womentowomen.com
The Women to Women Clinic in Yarmouth, Maine, focuses on treating women's health problems through education and participation. All practitioners at the Women to Women Clinic are trained in both traditional and functional medicine.

Nutrition

The George Mateljan Foundation

PO Box 25801
Seattle, WA 98165
www.whfoods.org
The George Mateljan Foundation is a nonprofit organization dedicated to making the world a healthier place by providing cutting-edge information about why the world's healthiest foods are the key to vibrant health and energy; and how you can easily make them a part of your healthy lifestyle.

Gut and Psychology Syndrome (GAPS) Diet

www.gutandpsychologysyndrome.com
The GAPS diet was developed by Dr. Natasha Campbell-McBride, a neurologist with a master's degree in nutrition. The diet focuses on the connection between the gut and the brain and describes how your food choices can affect your overall health.

Mark's Daily Apple

Mark Sisson
www.marksdailyapple.com
Mark Sisson is a former endurance athlete who uses his site, Mark's Daily Apple, to spread the latest research and information on living a Paleo lifestyle.

Specific Carbohydrate Diet (SCD) Lifestyle

Scdlifestyle.com
SCD Lifestyle was started by two friends who were able to correct their own health problems through proper diet, supplementation, and lifestyle changes. The founders provide regular nutrition and health information.

Appendix B: Glossary

Acid Reflux
A condition characterized by the backward flow (or reflux) of stomach contents into the esophagus

Acute
Abrupt onset

Amino Acids
Organic compounds that come together to form proteins

Antacids
Medications that neutralize stomach acid

Autoimmune Disease
An abnormal immune reaction in which the immune system attacks the body's own tissues

Bolus
A mass of chewed food in the mouth or digestive tract

Celiac Disease
A condition in which the ingestion of gluten triggers an immune response that attacks the lining of the small intestine

Chronic
Lasting for a long time or recurring

Chyme
The combination of partially digested food and gastric juices that passes from the stomach to the small intestine

Colitis
Inflammation of the mucosa (lining) of the colon

Constipation
Passage of small amounts of hard, dry bowel movements, usually fewer than three times a week

Crohn's Disease
A chronic inflammatory disease that most commonly affects the colon or the ileum

Diarrhea
Loose, watery stools that occur frequently

Digestion
Breaking down of food to simpler substances for absorption from the digestive system

Enzyme

A protein that speeds up chemical reactions and breaks down food into nutrients that the body can absorb

Essential Nutrients

Nutrients that your body requires but either cannot make or does not make in adequate amounts for proper health; you must consume these nutrients through the food you eat

Fiber

The part of a plant, such as cellulose, pectin, and lignan, that is not digested and helps to make stools bulky and soft

Food Allergy

An exaggerated IgE immune response triggered by a specific food

Food Intolerance

A nonallergic food reaction characterized by symptoms in one or more body systems

Food Sensitivity

An IgG immune response triggered by a specific food that is milder than a food allergy

Gluten

The protein component of wheat, barley, and rye

Gut

Refers to the stomach and intestines

Gut Flora

The good bacteria that naturally live in the intestines

H2 Receptor Antagonists

Medications that reduce the production of stomach acid by blocking histamine from reaching the parietal cells of the stomach

Heartburn

A burning sensation that radiates up from the stomach to the chest and throat

Hypochlorhydria

Low stomach acid

Inflammation

Redness, swelling, pain, and increased heat in a localized area of a tissue in response to injury or infection

Inflammatory Bowel Disease (IBD)

Chronic inflammation of all or part of the digestive tract

Irritable Bowel Syndrome (IBS)

A common functional bowel disorder causing abdominal pain, diarrhea, or constipation

Nonessential Nutrients

Nutrients that your body can make

Peristalsis
The involuntary muscular contractions responsible for moving materials through the digestive system

Probiotic
A substance that triggers the growth of beneficial bacteria in the gut

Proton Pump Inhibitors
Medications that reduce the body's production of stomach acid

Systemic
Widespread; relating to a whole system

Urticaria
Raised, itchy welts at the surface of the skin; hives

Standard U.S./Metric
Conversion Chart

VOLUME CONVERSIONS

U.S. Volume Measure	Metric Equivalent
⅛ teaspoon	0.5 milliliter
¼ teaspoon	1 milliliter
½ teaspoon	2 milliliters
1 teaspoon	5 milliliters
½ tablespoon	7 milliliters
1 tablespoon (3 teaspoons)	15 milliliters
2 tablespoons (1 fluid ounce)	30 milliliters
¼ cup (4 tablespoons)	60 milliliters
⅓ cup	90 milliliters
½ cup (4 fluid ounces)	125 milliliters
⅔ cup	160 milliliters
¾ cup (6 fluid ounces)	180 milliliters
1 cup (16 tablespoons)	250 milliliters
1 pint (2 cups)	500 milliliters
1 quart (4 cups)	1 liter (about)

WEIGHT CONVERSIONS

U.S. Weight Measure	Metric Equivalent
½ ounce	15 grams
1 ounce	30 grams
2 ounces	60 grams
3 ounces	85 grams
¼ pound (4 ounces)	115 grams
½ pound (8 ounces)	225 grams
¾ pound (12 ounces)	340 grams
1 pound (16 ounces)	454 grams

OVEN TEMPERATURE CONVERSIONS

Degrees Fahrenheit	Degrees Celsius
200 degrees F	95 degrees C
250 degrees F	120 degrees C
275 degrees F	135 degrees C
300 degrees F	150 degrees C
325 degrees F	160 degrees C
350 degrees F	180 degrees C
375 degrees F	190 degrees C
400 degrees F	205 degrees C
425 degrees F	220 degrees C
450 degrees F	230 degrees C

BAKING PAN SIZES

U.S.	Metric
8 × 1½ inch round baking pan	20 × 4 cm cake tin
9 × 1½ inch round baking pan	23 × 3.5 cm cake tin
11 × 7 × 1½ inch baking pan	28 × 18 × 4 cm baking tin
13 × 9 × 2 inch baking pan	30 × 20 × 5 cm baking tin
2 quart rectangular baking dish	30 × 20 × 3 cm baking tin
15 × 10 × 2 inch baking pan	30 × 25 × 2 cm baking tin (Swiss roll tin)
9 inch pie plate	22 × 4 or 23 × 4 cm pie plate
7 or 8 inch springform pan	18 or 20 cm springform or loose-bottom cake tin
9 × 5 × 3 inch loaf pan	23 × 13 × 7 cm or 2 lb narrow loaf or pâté tin
1½ quart casserole	1.5 liter casserole
2 quart casserole	2 liter casserole

Index